Pediatric Palliative

Pediatric Palliative Care: A Model for Exemplary Practice lays out a road map for health-care providers interested in optimizing care for seriously ill children and their families.

Grounded in clinical practice and the study of positive rather than problematic encounters between providers and parents, this book presents an evidence-based model of exemplary interaction. The chapters offer a clear understanding of the complex, holistic process of interaction between providers and parents, as well as the personal and professional knowledge and skills needed to interact in optimal ways.

This is a one-of-a-kind guidebook for health-care providers interested in (re)discovering how to maximize positive outcomes for both families and providers. It is also a valuable source of inspiration for educators, supervisors, and hospital administrators who want to facilitate personal and professional development and create supportive environments for students, providers, seriously ill children, and their families.

Betty Davies, MSN, PhD, is an adjunct professor in the School of Nursing, University of Victoria, British Columbia, Canada, and professor emerita in the Department of Family Health Care Nursing at the University of California, San Francisco, USA.

Rose Steele, RN, PhD, is a full professor in the School of Nursing, Faculty of Health, York University, Toronto, Ontario, Canada.

Jennifer Baird, RN, MPH, MSW, PhD, is the director of Clinical Services Education and Research at Children's Hospital Los Angeles, California, USA.

The Series in Death, Dying, and Bereavement

Series Editors: Robert A. Neimeyer, PhD, *Portland Institute for Loss and Transition, Oregon, USA,* and
Darcy L. Harris, PhD, *Western University Canada, Ontario, Canada*

Volumes published in the Series in Death, Dying, and Bereavement are representative of the multidisciplinary nature of the intersecting fields of death studies, suicidology, end-of-life care, and grief counseling. The series meets the needs of clinicians, researchers, paraprofessionals, pastoral counselors, and educators by providing cutting edge research, theory, and best practices on the most important topics in these fields—for today and for tomorrow.

Prescriptive Memories in Grief and Loss
The Art of Dreamscaping
Edited by Nancy Gershman and Barbara E. Thompson

Loss, Grief, and Attachment in Life Transitions
A Clinician's Guide to Secure Base Counseling
Jakob van Wielink, Leo Wilhelm, and Denise van Geelen-Merks

Non-Death Loss and Grief
Context and Clinical Implications
Edited by Darcy L. Harris

Superhero Grief
The Transformative Power of Loss
Edited by Jill A. Harrington and Robert A. Neimeyer

New Techniques of Grief Therapy
Bereavement and Beyond
Edited by Robert A. Neimeyer

Pediatric Palliative Care
A Model for Exemplary Practice
Betty Davies, Rose Steele, and Jennifer Baird

For more information about this series, please visit www.routledge.com/ Series-in-Death-Dying-and-Bereavement/book-series/SE0620.

Pediatric Palliative Care

A Model for Exemplary Practice

Betty Davies, Rose Steele, and Jennifer Baird

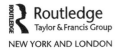

Routledge
Taylor & Francis Group

NEW YORK AND LONDON

First published 2022
by Routledge
605 Third Avenue, New York, NY 10158

and by Routledge
2 Park Square, Milton Park, Abingdon, Oxon, OX14 4RN

Routledge is an imprint of the Taylor & Francis Group, an informa business

Library of Congress Cataloging-in-Publication Data
Names: Davies, Betty, Ph. D. author. | Steele, Rose, author. | Baird,
    Jennifer (Nurse) author.
Title: Pediatric palliative care : a model for exemplary practice / Betty
    Davies, Rose Steele, Jennifer Baird.
Description: New York, NY : Routledge, 2021. | Series: Series in
    death, dying, and bereavement | Includes bibliographical references
    and index.
Identifiers: LCCN 2021029590 (print) | LCCN 2021029591 (ebook) |
    ISBN 9780367365684 (paperback) | ISBN 9780367365691
    (hardback) | ISBN 9780429352393 (ebook)
Subjects: LCSH: Terminally ill children—Care. | Children—Hospice care.
Classification: LCC RJ249 .D38 2021 (print) | LCC RJ249 (ebook) |
    DDC 618.92/0029—dc23
LC record available at https://lccn.loc.gov/2021029590
LC ebook record available at https://lccn.loc.gov/2021029591

ISBN: 978-0-367-36569-1 (hbk)
ISBN: 978-0-367-36568-4 (pbk)
ISBN: 978-0-429-35239-3 (ebk)

DOI: 10.4324/9780429352393

Typeset in Bembo
by Apex CoVantage, LLC

We dedicate this book to those health-care providers who consistently focus on what matters in the moment for children with life-threatening illness and their families.

Contents

Preface

The Background

When Betty's friend from childhood, Arlene, was a young mother of two preschool boys, she was diagnosed with stage 3 lymphoma. Over several years, Arlene endured total body radiation three times and countless rounds of chemotherapy. She turned out to be one of medicine's rare and celebrated miracles—she survived. Her experience with life-threatening illness taught Arlene that life is too short to not follow your dream. So she returned to school in midlife and became a much-acclaimed and award-winning artist.

During the years of Arlene's initial cancer experience, she often felt that the physicians related to her as just another source of data and many nurses treated her as just another patient on their day's to-do list. Certainly, she also encountered some very kind, thoughtful, and competent health-care professionals (HCPs), but they were comparatively few in number. Further, the distressing impact of the negative encounters remained among her worst memories of being so ill. Nearly 40 years later, Arlene was diagnosed in 2011 with pancreatic cancer. Despite her fears and trepidations, she chose to have chemotherapy once again, receiving treatment in the same hospital as before. But Arlene lamented that in the decades since she was last there, the treatments had become more complex, many tests were so much more complicated, and the equipment reminded her of a science fiction movie. Sadly, when it came to her as a person, nothing had changed for the better. She felt even more of an object in a much larger petri dish. All she wanted was for HCPs to remember that she was a human being inside the hospital gown.

Arlene's lament echoes in the comments we (the authors) continue to hear from many people about their contact with current health-care systems. In multiple research studies about parents' experiences in pediatric palliative care, whether or not directly asked about their encounters with pediatric health-care providers (PHCPs), parents inevitably talk about how important those exchanges are, particularly the negative ones that leave open wounds in their soul. One mother remained at the bedside of her child who had died about an hour before shift change. When making morning rounds, a new nurse poked her head into the room and, from the doorway, asked in a loud voice if Mrs. Clark knew that other children were waiting to be admitted. Another mother, Mrs. Ruiz, learned only during medical rounds that recent tests had confirmed her baby's life-threatening condition. The doctor did not tell her; she just overheard what he was saying to his colleagues. The impact of such encounters lingers in parents' hearts and minds forever. We find such stories professionally embarrassing at the very least, but they also affirm the goal that has motivated us during our careers: To make one of life's worst experiences—the serious illness and death of a loved one, particularly a child—as good as a bad experience can be or, at the very least, to not make such experiences even worse. Central to that goal is enhancing how HCPs relate to patients and their family members.

Betty's Story

I always wanted to be a nurse. My mother expressed surprise when I shared my earliest memory with her, because it was from when I was only 18 months old. I remembered being awake in the middle of night, sitting up in a hospital crib. I was hungry. A nursing sister (it was a Catholic hospital), silhouetted against the soft light of the hallway, appeared in the doorway and tiptoed to me. Somehow, she must have discovered why I was not sleeping. She left and I waited expectantly until she quickly and quietly returned, her arms crossed in the folds of her habit. Slowly, uncrossing her arms and like a magician wearing a cape, she produced a banana for me to eat. In recent years, I have wondered if that memory influenced my career choice—whether it did or not, I do believe that it imprinted in my mind an image of kindness in nurses.

As a young nursing student, therefore, I was eager to learn about Florence Nightingale, known as the Lady with the Lamp because of her kind and also meticulous caring for soldiers in military hospitals during the Crimean War. Of course, she was acclaimed for so much more, not just as the pioneer and founder of modern nursing but also as a reformer of the British military health-care system, hospitals, and public health. She was also respected for her knowledge of statistical analysis, philosophy, and spirituality—and all despite the social constraints on women at the time. "By any measure, she is one of the most towering figures in the Victorian age" (Dossey, 1999, p. vi).

Indeed, she was a visionary leader, so her words are worth heeding. In her *Notes on Nursing*, Nightingale (1860) put forward the fundamental principles of nursing, including that one purpose of nursing is to put the patient in the best condition for nature to act upon them. Putting the patient in the best condition requires that nurses do as Nightingale did: Create environments in which a nurse can integrate both art and science to become an instrument of healing. Throughout my nursing career as a clinician, a teacher, and a researcher, I have respected the competence of many nurses, physicians, and other HCPs, and I have been touched by the kindness shown by others. But

I still see a need for HCPs to place a greater emphasis on integrating both competence and kindness in creating environments conducive to healing in patients and their family members.

The course of my career was established early as a new second-year student and was motivated by my first experience with a patient's death. My patient assignment included Mrs. Jones, who was a middle-aged woman in the final stages of lung cancer. The night nurse reported surprise that Mrs. Jones had made it through the night. I said a silent prayer that she made it through the day! With trepidation, I approached Mrs. Jones' bedside only to discover that my prayer had not been answered. Our curriculum, similar to most professional education programs at the time, did not include any teaching about dying or death. I, therefore, took guidance from remembering a television show in which a patient died, and the nurse lowered the head of the bed and drew the curtain. I then anxiously reported to the charge nurse that Mrs. Jones had died. While engaged in a phone conversation with the pharmacy, the charge nurse simply pointed to the shelf of resource books and whispered that the procedure book was there, which translated into me looking up the procedure for caring for a body after death and following it. I recognized that she was coping with too few staff to care for too many seriously ill patients, but at the same time her abrupt and detached reaction compounded my personal trauma of carrying out this procedure for the first time. This experience, along with numerous others that followed, sowed seeds of curiosity about death and how nurses and other HCPs promoted healing for those who were facing death or who were grieving.

In pediatrics, I learned that most parents, understandably, lacked skill in explaining diagnoses of serious illness to their ill children or to siblings. Similarly, most PHCPs were challenged when facing a death or with offering healing words to grieving parents and children. But the importance of such encounters was emphasized in my doctoral dissertation about bereaved siblings for whom the central factor affecting their grief reactions was the nature of their encounters with PHCPs and other significant adults in their lives. Only a few adults really listened to them; other adults' lack of any conversation at all or their insensitive comments only added to siblings' hurt, confusion about what was happening, sense of not belonging, and feeling as if, in their parents' eyes, they no longer mattered as much as the brother or sister who had died. In my program of research about the experiences of diverse types of families in palliative care, participants noted that even though some clinicians were caring or human, others seemed programmed to follow procedures or were detached like scientists. A common source of distress was HCPs whose professionalism interfered with their capacity to act like human beings.

When a child or adult was seriously ill or dying, "human" exchanges with care providers clearly created a supportive environment in which the synthesis of both science and art determined patients and their family members' perceptions of quality of care and healing outcomes. Yet, despite this understanding, PHCPs knew relatively little about what facilitates the human aspect of encounters between providers and those for whom they care. The study upon which this book is based was designed to address this question.

As a teacher in a variety of educational programs and settings, the human aspect of faculty–student interaction also stood out for me as being critical to students' learning. I witnessed teachers who created environments conducive to students' healing and learning, but I also saw too many situations in which the human aspect was ignored or forgotten. How do educators expect students to learn to care for patients as whole persons if their teachers do not model that role with them? The same can be said for administrator–staff interactions.

In the latter part of my career, I experienced the joy of having my former students become current colleagues in our shared journey toward humanizing health care. This is especially true for Rose and Jenni, whom I welcome wholeheartedly as co-authors of this book.

Rose's Story

I have had an eclectic career in which relationships between HCPs and patients/families have been central from the beginning, though increasingly so as I developed professionally and matured personally. After my initial hospital training as a registered nurse in Scotland, I worked in an adult surgical unit and then moved into intensive care areas. When I immigrated to Canada, I continued my clinical practice in adult critical care areas, both medical and surgical, for another 15 years. Too often I found myself frustrated by colleagues who did not listen to patients or who refused to allow a family member to assist in basic care for a patient. I struggled when, in my opinion, colleagues disempowered patients and families, and I also faced colleagues' displeasure at times when I wanted to work with patients and families. For example, when a patient was on a ventilator, I might invite a relative to be with me during the bedbath and to help in whatever way was possible, but some colleagues chastised me for my actions even though I could see the positive benefits to both patient and family. I will never forget the man with amyotrophic lateral sclerosis whose only piece of control was to let us know when he wanted to be suctioned—yet some colleagues refused his request and would only suction him on their schedule. I learned that the golden rule "Do to others what you would want done to you" is not useful in health care. Rather, the golden rule should be "Do to others what they want done to them." A subtle difference in some ways perhaps, but I found that it made the world of difference to patients and their families.

As I continued my education, I was introduced to the principles of palliative care and suddenly I felt more at home. Working with patients and families instead of doing things to them, listening to what they wanted, and doing my best to facilitate what was needed all felt like such a good fit for me. I began to conduct research in the area of adult palliative care, but I found that even when patients and families were clear on what they needed (and did not need), some HCPs were unable to understand. Instead, these providers would say that patients/families just needed more information or that they did not really know what they needed, and it was the HCP's role to do what the provider thought was best. I continued to wonder what it was that made HCPs more open to what patients/families wanted.

In my PhD program, I became involved with Betty as her research assistant in an evaluation of a children's hospice and as her supervisee. I had not worked in pediatrics other than in my initial education, and as a mother I did not want to conduct research with families whose child was dying. But over a few months, the parents on our research team persuaded me that they needed someone to provide a voice because nobody really understood their lives. They told me they would help me understand so I could help other HCPs who, in turn, would help families. So began my journey into pediatric palliative care. I also continued with my adult research until about 2009 and then concentrated only on pediatric palliative care.

Whether adult medicine, surgery, or intensive care, adult oncology palliative care, or pediatric palliative care, I was still confronted by HCPs who related to patients and families in ways that seemed less than optimal. Often the care was good, but I was learning of ways to make it even better. I was intrigued when Betty talked about results from other studies she had done and how she was hearing similar things—that only some HCPs were excellent. I too wanted to know exactly what it was that enabled some HCPs to engage in excellent ways. The study described in this book, along with all of the combined previous research, teaching, and clinical work that Betty, Jenni, and I have done, is our way of helping HCPs optimally engage with patients and families so that all concerned have positive outcomes.

Jenni's Story

I became a nurse after completing undergraduate and graduate degrees in clinical social work. My nursing practice is, therefore, informed and enriched by my social work background, which includes a commitment to social justice and a person-in-environment orientation that focuses my understanding of individuals within the context of their family, friends, and community. My social work training encompassed a broad range of experiences, from case management in an urban homeless day shelter to special education eligibility assessment for children receiving early intervention services. As a practicing social worker, I facilitated communication skill-building groups for families of children experiencing behavioral challenges in school. In each of these experiences, I was challenged to understand life experiences far different from my own and to bridge those differences, thus establishing a therapeutic connection to facilitate service delivery. The clients with whom I worked—whether an older woman experiencing chronic homelessness and an exacerbation of schizophrenia or the couple unable to help their son control his behavior in the classroom setting—taught me the value of authentic engagement and the power of careful listening to others' stories, skills that have served me well in my nursing career and that, unfortunately, are too infrequently practiced in many health-care settings.

The majority of my clinical practice as a nurse has been in the pediatric intensive care unit (PICU) where I worked closely with, and on behalf of, families in crisis due to the severity of their child's illness. Within my first week after orientation as a new graduate nurse, five children died in the PICU. I quickly learned that pediatric end-of-life care was imperfect, at times haphazard, and offered inconsistent support to families as it was rife with conflicting opinions and poor-quality communication. I spent many night shifts in the PICU standing vigil with parents, worried that we as a health-care team had not adequately prepared them for what was to come. Dissatisfaction with this reality drove me to return to school in search of the tools that would allow me to investigate better ways of delivering nursing care to dying children and their families.

Along the path of my nursing doctoral studies and guided by insights from my work with Betty, I came to realize that the poor communication I observed in the end-of-life period was a symptom of a much larger problem that was not unique to the end of life. Indeed, the haphazard nature of care for dying children was the natural consequence of systems poorly designed to understand and accommodate the individual experiences of families all along the care trajectory, from the time of diagnosis until the end of life. My current work is, therefore, focused on developing systems that are responsive to individual family needs, which begins with an understanding of how to help clinicians engage authentically and offer support to fully honor and embrace each family's unique experiences.

Our Shared Story

The three of us share a common view that connections or human relationships between HCPs and patients/family members are crucial to humanizing health care. We have learned that when encounters do not go well—for example, when providers are rude, do not listen, or disregard patients' or family members' requests or needs for information, comfort, and hope—individuals suffer unnecessarily from memories that cause distress long into the future. In contrast, when encounters are human, then family members carry memories that lend strength for healing. Reassuringly, patients and parents and other family members report that most HCPs are okay or good at what they do and that they are generally satisfied with the overall care that they and their loved ones have received. However, they also report that some providers are not so good, and they provide details of distressing encounters. Only a few HCPs are described as excellent, defined as the ones who treat them like a human being. We were left asking: Should it not be the goal for all HCPs to engage with patients/family members so that they all feel that they are being treated as human beings? Thus, in the study that gave rise to this book, we focused on positive interactions between PHCPs and parents to learn what made it possible for some, but not all, PHCPs to be perceived by others as excellent or human.

We share a widespread concern that health care today is dehumanizing due to such factors as advances in technology, treatments, and interventions, reliance on procedures and protocols, ever-expanding bureaucracy, and an emphasis on professionalization and standardization. In response to this trend of depersonalizing health care, some authors have sought to improve communication, but often this attempt has resulted in communication strategies being taught and practiced more as procedures or protocols. The result is often a narrow focus on various techniques or strategies for engaging in difficult topics such as giving bad news. Others have attempted to counteract dehumanization in health care by developing concepts of patient-centered care, individualized care, family-centered care, relational care, and narrative medicine—concepts that promote or advocate for a different kind of health care. However, we have noted that each of these concepts has its own adherents who, despite their common purpose and commonalities, rarely acknowledge the others. Thus, we believe that an overall change must happen in conceptualizing what is required of HCPs in relating to patients and families.

Focus of the Book

In this book, we offer a new evidence-based conceptualization and model that we believe can guide understanding of and learning about what is necessary for PHCPs to engage authentically during interaction with patients/family members and also with their colleagues. We believe our book accomplishes what others do not. Many books on communication focus on the idea of HCPs applying what they learn to do and say to patients with the goal of somehow changing them (the patients), rather than recognizing that providers must focus on what they themselves bring to the situation. Our conceptualization provides support for the concepts of patient- or family-centered, individualized, and relational care, as well as narrative medicine: Proponents of these concepts advocate for behaviors that we found are evident in PHCPs' exemplary encounters with others. The model emphasizes the complexity of human-to-human interaction, regardless of discipline. It incorporates principles of communication and depends not only upon the firm foundation provided by personal factors but also upon a broad worldview, values of equity, family-centered care, and integrity, as well as a commitment to authentic engagement.

Exemplary pediatric health-care providers (EPPs) engage in direct care activities, in connecting behaviors, and in the process of exquisitely attuning to particularities of the situation in the moment, resulting in a milieu of mattering that leads to positive outcomes for both themselves and parents. EPPs are also grounded in their work team and setting, and they are aware of the pressures exerted by contextual aspects of the institution and societal trends and values. By focusing on what EPPs do well, findings of our study showed that not only is it possible for PHCPs to practice in this way but those who do are recognized as being the best at what they do. Moreover, the conceptualization shows that meaningful connections are not just a matter of personality or temperament as is often claimed but <u>can</u> and <u>must</u> be learned.

This book is unique in its use of the metaphor of a prairie windmill. Metaphors increase attention, leading to both a deeper processing and a better recall of the material. The windmill metaphor helps to provide conceptual clarity, which, in turn, helps PHCPs envision the whole of authentic engagement while seeing the interdependence and simultaneity of the various components. Naming the components provides words for both PHCPs and patients/family members to describe explicitly what EPPs do to engage in exemplary interactions and, thus, identify the specific components that may need to be reinforced or strengthened while teaching, mentoring, or supervising PHCPs and students. Overall, the metaphor helps us to achieve our ultimate goal of providing meaningful guidance about how PHCPs can succeed in connecting with and respecting patients, their family members, students, and colleagues as whole persons, thereby humanizing health care.

Content of the Book

A central characteristic of EPPs was that they intentionally engaged in all components of exemplary interaction at all times—that is, they consistently engaged in the whole of interaction. To remain true to this significant finding, we were motivated to describe the conceptualization in a book rather than in a series of papers in professional journals that would necessitate breaking down the whole into segments that are published in a disconnected manner. We want to help readers develop a broader perspective on EPP interaction by demonstrating that <u>all</u> components of our model are required, that there is a need to see the whole, and that clinicians need to learn about themselves before they can effectively engage with others in human-to-human interaction that embodies ethical practice and family-centered care.

We read and critiqued more than a dozen books that seemed to align with our book. However, they tended to be specific to a particular discipline, and most aimed to improve communication in health care through the teaching of techniques and protocols rather than by focusing on how to achieve authentic engagement with patients and families. We envision our book being used in educational settings as complementary to some of the existing textbooks, as well as in clinical settings for clinicians' ongoing professional development. The research team and the research participants who developed the model of authentic engagement were from a range of health-care professions. Thus, the book is relevant across disciplines, so any provider whose discipline includes interaction with patients—for example, nursing, social work, medicine, psychology, occupational therapy, respiratory therapy, and chaplaincy—can find utility in our conceptualization.

We intend this book for all who are interested in or actively responsible for teaching and supervising health-care students about what to strive for in themselves so as to engage authentically with patients/family members and with colleagues. The book is also for practicing clinicians who are eager to find a new way of understanding and explaining the complexity of the seemingly simple activity of engaging with all those with whom they work. It is applicable too for administrators who have the authority to implement changes that will create environments that support providers in their practice.

Outline of Content

We aim to optimize interaction between and among PHCPs and those whom they serve. In the first two chapters, we provide background to the study and a brief overview of the model. In the subsequent chapters, we then discuss various aspects of the model in some detail, though always emphasizing the importance of the whole, as it is the synthesizing of all aspects that results in optimal interaction. We include questions and ideas to raise readers' awareness and to facilitate thinking about their own worldview, values, commitment, and practice because it is important to recognize that HCPs bring themselves as persons, not just their professional roles, to every encounter. We also show that interaction is influenced by teamwork, the culture of the clinical setting and the institution, and the larger society within which all encounters occur. Finally, we discuss the milieu of mattering and the outcomes that result from the model, as well as the implications of using our model.

To protect the identity of parents or PHCPs cited in the quotes, epigraphs, and examples, we use pseudonyms and the singular "they," and alter personal details. Some quotes and examples are actually compilations from multiple people who represent a variety of clinical settings and disciplines. They were carefully compiled to allow the reader to reflect on professional interactions across the lifespan and throughout the wide spectrum of environments in which care is delivered.

In sharing our ideas, our research findings, and our experiences with you, our readers, our hope is that you will find them useful in your own work with patients and their family members, with students, and with peers. We hope that this book not only offers you an intriguing perspective on PHCP interaction but also inspires you to strengthen or reinstate your commitment to authentic engagement—that initial desire to help others and to make a difference in the lives of those who are vulnerable, the motivation that brought you into health care in the first place.

References

Dossey, B. M. (1999). *Florence nightingale: Mystic, visionary, healer.* Springhouse Corporation.

Nightingale, F. (1860). *Notes on nursing.* D. Appleton & Co.

Series Editors' Foreword

In 2003, David Kuhl introduced readers to the voices of the palliative patients that he interviewed at the end of their lives, providing unique insights into what patients and their families wanted their health-care providers to know. Many of the patient interviewees expressed gratitude for the care that they had received during their time in palliative care. However, there were also candid accounts of missed opportunities and even harm patients described that occurred not from their disease but from how some of their health-care providers responded to them. These descriptions led Kuhl to use the phrase iatrogenic trauma (Kuhl, 2003), meaning pain and suffering patients experienced that were created by their encounters with the health-care system.

In *Pediatric Palliative Care: A Model for Exemplary Practice*, the authors step forward from earlier writings about patient experiences into the world of pediatric palliative care, observing and interviewing parents as well as the health-care providers about their experiences. We are reminded of the very complex and potentially overwhelming world that parents and their sick children must navigate during an incredibly stressful time. Pediatric palliative health-care providers are uniquely situated to care for these families with compassion, with the hope of fostering a sense of respect, feeling cared about (*mattering*), and feeling empowered as much as possible. These parents are hurting. They are grieving the losses associated with their child's critical and complex illness, including the loss of their hopes, dreams, and desires for the future. In essence, they are living through a parent's worst nightmare. The sensitivity and compassion associated with exemplary care is a salve to this deeply painful wound.

But what exactly is exemplary care? How is it different from routine care? How can exemplary care be enhanced? These are the questions that the authors asked, and the answers to these questions and many others can be found here. What the authors do in this book is to break down what it means to provide not just good care but exceptional care to these families, offering snippets from the voices of parents, descriptions of exceptional care when it was observed, and reflections of the exemplary care providers themselves. The exploration of exactly what constitutes exemplary care is practical; readers will find a treasure trove of suggestions, ways to explore attitudes that enhance care provision and to develop deeper understandings about the impact of structural, systemic, and interactional components upon care delivery. There is no stone unturned; there is practical wisdom about self-awareness and self-reflection, and there is also an in-depth discussion about the influence of external factors such as team dynamics, the institutional milieu, social attitudes about death, and how social justice and diversity issues are experienced by pediatric patients and their families.

A foundational theme throughout the book is the importance of shared experiences between families and health-care providers. Parents and their children are identified as the crucial members of the health-care team and not peripheral to planned interventions. Rather than simply being a vehicle for the transmission of information, communication becomes a valued shared experience, where ideas are exchanged and deep listening to parents situates their voice as the primary guide for the health-care providers.

In a world where much of the essence of being human in health care gets lost in the technology and the objectification of both care providers and the recipients of that care, this book provides a breath of fresh air, reminding us that it is the relationships that we form with others that matter, and caring relationships within the context of a very painful time matter even more.

Darcy Harris
Series Co-editor

Reference

Kuhl, D. (2003). *What dying people want: Practical wisdom for the end of life*. Anchor Canada.

Acknowledgments

Gratitude is a memory of the heart.

Massieu

Betty has long valued this quotation that so simply describes the nature of gratitude. We wish to express our appreciation to the many individuals who, from the start of the research project from which this book evolved, have provided us with so many "memories of the heart."

We owe sincere gratitude to the members of the project's research team. Heartfelt thanks to our co-investigators—Hal Siden, Susan Albersheim, Caron Strahlendorf, Susan Cadell, and Gweneth Doane—who contributed to data analysis meetings, always showing enthusiasm for the project while asking astute questions. Hal, Susan, and Caron also expertly guided the study through institutional ethics review and monitored the study progress at their respective sites.

With diligence and enthusiasm our research coordinators, first Anne-Mette Hermansen and then Michelle Biferie, kept track of not only the project's progress but also the people involved, which was sometimes a challenge given our multidisciplinary study included researchers from four academic institutions and three clinical settings located within two health-care institutions. They also assisted with some data collection and contributed to our analysis discussions. The bulk of data collection was in the skillful hands of our research nurse, Deepshikha Garga, and our research assistant, Yuan Zhao. Dee and Yuan enthusiastically engaged in the day-to-day practicalities of recruitment and data collection; they also provided insights into the data analysis, in particular about their own cultures and traditions, all of which proved to be invaluable.

We also appreciate the practical contributions of Kortney Story, who, with impressive speed and accuracy, transcribed the vast majority of our interviews. Michael Jew, a medical work-study student, and Jenni Baird, then a doctoral student, offered valuable insights from their individual clinical perspectives.

Last but definitely not least of the research team members was Guenther Krueger who most competently served as our research analyst for this qualitative study. In his innovative role, he contributed his extensive knowledge about the NVivo data management software program and was integral to the process of analysis—consistently competent, comprehensive, and cheerful in his many contributions. Further, Guenther's insights on an earlier draft of the book were vital to the final product.

Our research team members brought experience from nursing, medicine, social work, counseling, anthropology, sociology, and public health that resulted in valuable disciplinary insights, as well as theoretical and clinical expertise, that enhanced and expanded data analysis in ways that would not have been possible from a unitary disciplinary perspective. Moreover, during the course of the research project, our core team experienced numerous life crises and transitions—pregnancies, marriages, divorces, deaths of family members and other loved ones, moving, illnesses among team members and their families. Each of these experiences caused a ripple in our progress, but we were never stymied—with support for and patience with one another, we forged ahead. We are so grateful for everyone's contributions to making our team strong, collaborative, and caring.

To Greg Glover, a very grateful thank you for his excellent artwork for various presentations and also for this book. He was able to magically convert our rudimentary sketches of our ideas into representative images. We are especially grateful for his most welcome assistance with our windmill photograph, saving Jenni a second hike to recapture another photograph, and with translating technical requirements into reality.

This project would never have been possible without the acceptance, support, and guidance from key physicians, nurses, administrators, and parents at the sites where the study was conducted: Filomena Nalewajek, Tanice Miller, Janie Burns, Kerry Keats, Sharon Rai, John Gojevic, and Monty Armstrong from the children's hospice; Linda Dix-Cooper, Jennifer Claydon, and Brian Lupton from the neonatal intensive care unit (NICU); and Cindy Stutzer, Agnes Pietrowski, Dan Mornar, and Susan Greig from oncology. These individuals introduced the study to families initially, facilitated meetings between the researchers and the health-care providers in each site, and served as members of our Clinician Advisory Group or our Parent Advisory Group. We also extend our thanks to all the other health-care providers and parents who served in advisory capacities, providing consultation as a group or individually as needed.

We so appreciate the parents and health-care providers who consented to talk with us and to permit us to observe their interactions—without them there would have been no project. We especially appreciate their eagerness to talk thoughtfully and openly about their experiences. We hope that our questions and observations in their daily lives were not too burdensome, and we are so grateful that many of them have told us that our findings were worth their time and effort. In addition, we have had numerous opportunities to share these research findings with other parents, family members, and professional health-care providers through conferences, workshops, and other presentations. To all the individuals in those many organizations who have facilitated this process, we also extend our gratitude.

This research project was initially conceived while Betty was at the University of California San Francisco (UCSF). Thank you to all those wonderful health-care providers at UCSF Children's Hospital, particularly Robin Kramer, Anu Banerjee, Sally Sehring, and Colin Partridge, who eagerly contributed to the development of the first pilot study, and to Guenther, who in his desire for an opportunity to be involved in research traveled to San Francisco to help with the pilot study. Thanks also to Sharon Kaufman whose consultation about ethnographic grounded theory was exceptionally helpful. Betty then accepted a position in Canada, where, with the aid of a Research Facilitation Grant from the University of Victoria, she conducted a second pilot study in Vancouver. The full project was then made possible by funding from the Canadian Institutes of Health Research (Grant # MOP-115009), for which we are extremely grateful. We also acknowledge the generous support that Rose received through York University.

We are extremely grateful to Anna Moore, senior editor with Routledge, for believing in this project from the start and for her thoughtful guidance, kind assistance, and prompt attention to our every query throughout the publishing process. We feel very fortunate to have worked with an editor as insightful and punctual. We are also thankful to the series editors, Bob Neimeyer and Darcy Harris, who welcomed our book in their series.

Betty's heart is filled with gratitude for her friends, family, and colleagues who offered steady encouragement throughout the research project and the writing of this book. It takes a village to not only raise a child but also sustain them as adults through life! A particular thanks to Joanne Reimer and Chuck Corr for offering to read the entire manuscript in attempts to create an appropriate title for the book. Finally, Betty's deepest gratitude goes to her husband, Tom Attig, who helped her in too many ways to enumerate—for always being there, for making her laugh, for helping her think, for practical advice and encouragement, and for celebrating each phase of the project and this book. His presence in Betty's life is proof that miracles do happen.

Finally, as partners in writing this book, we will not soon forget our biweekly Friday Zoom meetings and our days-long, in-person meetings around Betty's dining room table. Our discussions sparked streams of ideas and insights, interspersed with gales of laughter—a perfect combination for creativity, camaraderie, and collaboration. Our friendship will continue even though this book is complete.

About the Authors

Betty Davies, MSN, PhD, is an adjunct professor in the School of Nursing, University of Victoria, Victoria, British Columbia, Canada, and Professor Emerita in Family Health Care Nursing, University of California San Francisco, San Francisco, USA. Her long career has focused on palliative/ hospice care for adults and children and their families, the impact of palliative care on health-care providers, and palliative care education. Her extensive research is reported in nearly 200 articles and book chapters, and two books: *Fading Away: The Experience of Transition in Families Facing Terminal Illness* and *Shadows in the Sun: Experiences of Sibling Bereavement in Childhood*. Dr. Davies is co-founder of Canuck Place, North America's first free-standing children's hospice. She serves on the editorial board of several significant journals and is the recipient of numerous awards for her contributions as a clinician, researcher, and teacher, most notably the University of Alberta Alumni Honor Award and the Pediatric Award of Excellence from the Pediatric Network of Palliative Care for Children and the Canadian Hospice and Palliative Care Association.

Rose Steele, RN, PhD, is a professor in the School of Nursing, Faculty of Health, York University in Toronto, Ontario, Canada. She was initially a nurse who practiced in adult settings only, but over the past 20+ years, since she was introduced to pediatric palliative care, her research has shifted to focus on this important but under-researched field. Dr. Steele has used both qualitative and quantitative approaches during her research as she chooses the method that best helps her answer the research question. She has also conducted research in the area of adult oncology. Since 1996, Dr. Steele has been the PI, Co-PI, or Co-I on 30 external grants that were awarded a total of over $4.3 million. She has published 12 refereed book chapters and almost 50 articles, as well as presented over 90 conference papers plus 40 posters.

Jennifer Baird, RN, MPH, MSW, PhD, is Director, Clinical Services Education and Research at Children's Hospital, Los Angeles, California, USA. Her research focuses on the family's experience of pediatric care delivery systems, with an emphasis on the ways in which interactions among providers and families impact patient safety and families' perceptions of care. Her experience as a pediatric nurse in acute and critical care settings, combined with training in social work, public health, and health services research methodologies, informs this work. Dr. Baird has a current grant from the Lucile Packard Foundation for Children's Health to study changes in the quality of discharge care for hospitalized patients through the use of a learning collaborative, and she serves as a collaborator on a Patient-Centered Outcomes Research Institute-funded study of a family-centered, rounds-based communication intervention. She has published 17 peer-reviewed articles and presented 20 conference papers.

Boxes, Figures, and Tables

Boxes

Figures

Tables

Abbreviations

CCC: Complex, chronic, and potentially life-threatening condition
EPP: Exemplary pediatric health-care provider
HCP: Health-care professional
NICU: Neonatal intensive care unit
PHCP: Pediatric health-care provider
PICU: Pediatric intensive care unit
SI: Symbolic interactionism

1 Introduction to Interaction

Through her tears, Maria Gonzales, a Mexican American mother of a baby diagnosed prenatally with a life-threatening genetic condition, recounted her humiliation and exasperation when she was in her 16th hour of labor that had begun earlier than expected. Maria spoke very little English and had no family available to accompany her to the hospital. Her husband, who was also her interpreter, was working out of town, and, though he was trying to get to the hospital, he had not yet arrived. A young female physician had stood at the doorway of the labor room, coffee in one hand and a donut in the other, and called out cheerfully: Still waiting? Hang in there! Maria had no idea what the doctor meant by still waiting. Waiting for what? Was there something she was supposed to do and was that the reason no one was with her or paying attention to her? Maria heard the words "hang in there" but did not understand the meaning of this common colloquialism. Instead of being reassured as the doctor may have intended, Maria's fear was enhanced by her confusion about what it was she herself was supposed to be doing. Moreover, Maria had never experienced a professional eating casually while with a patient, and in her culture to do so was considered very rude. In recounting this encounter three years later, Maria cried again, still troubled by the memory of feeling so alone, so helpless, so confused, and so ignored by this physician.

Maria Gonzales' experience illustrates what we (the authors) know from our own work in the field of pediatric palliative care along with two decades of literature focused on families of children with complex, chronic, and potentially life-threatening conditions (CCCs), which are conditions that affect multiple organ and body systems, are long term, and carry the potential of early death (Feudtner et al., 2000). The stress of constant worry and the uncertainty of their child's prognosis permeates the lives of these parents, and they deserve optimal sensitivity from those who care for their child and them. Insensitive interactions with pediatric health-care providers (PHCPs) threaten these parents' well-being; their sense of security, comfort, and capability to care for their child; their perceptions of the quality of care their child and they receive; their trust in the health-care system and in PHCPs; how they cope with their child's illness over the long term; and the course of bereavement if and when their child dies (Butler et al., 2015; Cadell et al., 2014; Davies et al., 2007; Melin-Johansson et al., 2014; Stevenson et al., 2013; Xafis et al., 2015).

DOI: 10.4324/9780429352393-1

Supportive and human-to-human interaction may be especially important for non–English-speaking and socially and economically disadvantaged families, such as Maria Gonzales and her family, a crucial consideration as population demographics shift due to immigration and socioeconomic changes (Contro et al., 2010; Davies et al., 2011). For example, training programs for ethnically Chinese volunteers and caregivers have identified the importance of skilled interactions within a medical setting as a priority for optimal interpersonal strategies for conveying end-of-life information to this particular population (Chou et al., 2008; Munet-Vilaro, 2004). In addition, attention should be paid to potential gender and role differences because fathers report that they receive less attention than mothers and have their own unique experiences to share (Davies et al., 2004, 2013). Evidence suggests that parents who perceive PHCPs as impersonal and uncaring experience guilt long after their child's death when they feel they were not given information in a dignified way, cannot discuss their child's condition with staff, and have unanswered questions (Davies et al., 2010; Surkan et al., 2006).

Parents' worries about their child's care are typically centered on negative or unhelpful interactions. They express feelings of anger and frustration when PHCPs fail to respond appropriately, as illustrated by parents' distress when PHCPs are rude, dismissive of their observations about their child, or treat their children as guinea pigs rather than as human beings (Contro et al., 2002; Davies et al., 2013; Woodgate, 2006). Parents resent being made to feel inadequate in their parenting role, being pushed aside, or being ignored as busy PHCPs go about their routine work. Without sufficient ongoing emotional and social support, parents feel isolated and distressed (Contro et al., 2004). Some parents even advise that PHCPs need specific interpersonal skills training (Garwick et al., 1998).

The Power of Negative Interactions

Given the impact of parents' encounters with insensitive PHCPs, it is not surprising that parents focus on their negative interactions. Nor is it surprising that researchers address problems identified by parents or other groups of people and that clinicians are often problem-focused. As nurses ourselves, we understand the desire of PHCPs to seek ways to address the difficult situations they confront every day, for example, telling parents of their child's cancer diagnosis. We acknowledge that clinicians want to know what to say; they want to learn how to find the right words to inform, teach, and comfort. There is a need (and a responsibility) to know how to do such things. However, this basic, sometimes desperate, need is often based on the idea that for every problem there is an answer in the form of an action or procedure that, if implemented, will guide clinicians to successful resolution of the problem. Moreover, because health care is a fast-paced world in which efficiency is the hallmark of success, clinicians sometimes mistakenly believe that if they can identify the problem and know what to say, then they can follow the procedure quickly and check off that the problem has been solved. Thus, clinicians have a tendency to focus on problems.

In a classic psychology article, Baumeister and colleagues (2001) extensively reviewed the evidence pertaining to the general hypothesis that bad is stronger than good. They concluded that the idea is a basic and wide-ranging principle across a broad range of psychological phenomena found in everyday events, including major life events (e.g., trauma), close relationship outcomes, social network patterns, interpersonal interactions, and learning processes. They suggested that the comparative strength of a bad perspective reflects an evolutionary adaptive mechanism, because negative experiences often motivate human beings to change, to seek alternative ways of doing things or thinking about what they do.

We know from psychology, and from our own experiences, that people can often remember the details of negative experiences much more than the details of positive experiences. For example, when people are asked where they or their family members were on the day that the World Trade Center in New York City was attacked, most people can repeat details of the day—not only where they were, but also what exactly they were doing just before they heard the news reports. This remarkable ability to conjure up even the smallest details surrounding a tragic or traumatic event is directly related to the intensity of the event itself. In other words, the more emotionally disturbing the experience is, the more likely people are to commit it to memory, because memory and emotion are inextricably linked in the human brain. In her book, *The Balance Within: The Science Connecting Health and Emotions*, Dr. Esther Sternberg (2001) pointed out that memory is one of the major factors mediating between sensation and emotional experience. She proposed that memories of past experience become triggers for future psycho-emotional responses and so influence the present experience. Thus, when parents have had a negative experience with a PHCP, recounting that event can continue to trigger negative emotional responses. The parents' memories become entrenched with the negative emotions associated with them.

Moreover, Dr. Bessell van der Kolk, a professor of psychiatry at Boston University Medical School and a leading researcher in the area of traumatic stress, claimed that stress occurring at the hands of people who are supposed to take care of you is particularly traumatic because one's sense of safety and predictability is threatened (van der Kolk, 2015). Parents of children with CCCs are, of course, already feeling vulnerable and lost in the uncertainty that characterizes their situation. Having negative interactions with professionals, the very people from whom parents expect help, only magnifies the distress they already feel.

Baumeister et al. (2001) further reported that bad impressions and bad stereotypes are quicker to form and are more resistant to disconfirmation than are good ones. Moreover, the initial acts in an interaction create expectancies and set the tone for further ones, and if subsequent acts differ, then the expectancies are violated. Therefore, if a PHCP starts off by behaving in a friendly, interested manner and then becomes aloof and unfriendly, the impact on the patient or family member is greater than if a practitioner is initially aloof and unfriendly and then warms up. Violations of expected behavior produce strong reactions, but violations in the negative direction have even stronger effects than a positive direction. Furthermore, Gottman (1994, as cited in Baumeister et al., 2001) reported that bad events are so much stronger than good ones that the good must far outnumber the bad in order to prevail. Gottman's index (1994, as cited in Baumeister et al., 2001) suggests that bad events are on average five times as powerful as good ones, at least with regard to relationships, such as the personal relationships between parents and PHCPs. Thus, to compensate for every negative interaction with one PHCP, parents must experience five positive ones from the same provider. Given the large number of staff that parents and their ill children encounter in hospital, the likelihood may be low for opportunities that provide the requisite number of compensatory interactions from any one provider.

Communication versus Interaction

Because negative PHCP–parent interactions are so powerful and influential, we therefore understood why so much has been written about relationships that were not good or interactions that did not go well. Further, it became clear why very little had been written about interactions that had gone well, despite the emphasis on communication skills in professional education. A vast literature that stresses the importance of clinicians' effective communication with families of patients nearly always highlights problems in communication. These problems include avoidance of discussions regarding care and prognosis, missed opportunities for conversation, and a failure of open, thoughtful, supportive, and hopeful dialogue so that, consequently, parents' opinions and personhood are ignored (Heller & Solomon, 2005). Even curricula (e.g., American Association of Colleges of Nursing, 2018; National Hospice and Palliative Care Organization, 2018) and training workshops (Kolarik et al., 2006) specifically designed to enhance excellence in pediatric palliative care often fail to address issues of optimal interaction within their communication skills training modules. Areas of concern are typically restricted to "how to" guidelines for giving bad news, helping to make decisions, and employing active listening skills rather than developing an understanding of the broader concepts of interaction (Contro et al., 2002). Such guidelines imply that providing information is the central aspect of communication between PHCPs and parents, with the result that communication is often perceived simply as another procedure or protocol to follow rather than as a component of a complex relationship between individuals.

But we also knew that parents consistently identify valued interaction patterns, such as when PHCPs give basic information and explain the implications of the information while also attending to the questions and emotional responses of parents and children (Davies et al., 2010). In addition to clinical competence, parents value how PHCPs interact with, relate to, and form human–human relationships with them (Steele & Davies, 2006; Woodgate, 2006). Fathers have commented that most interactions are good, with some not-so-good, but there are only a few that are excellent (Davies & Gudmundsdottir, 2006). The excellent interactions stood out because those PHCPs listened to the fathers, sat down when they talked to them, looked them in the eye, did not treat the children like guinea pigs, and regarded fathers as human beings. Parents also value small acts of human kindness (Macdonald et al., 2005), as well as support, assistance, and empathy (Janzen et al., 2003–2004; Rehm, 1999). They recognize the emotional impact of interactions with PHCPs and the importance of collaboration and partnership but lament that finding true partnerships is not easy (Bonanno et al., 2005). In contrast to their detailed descriptions of what went wrong in a negative interaction, parents often have difficulty articulating what enables PHCPs to provide exceptional care. They generally refer to nonspecific supportive qualities, including a parent–professional alliance that captures elements of trust, respect, commitment, care, compassion, continuity, and community, as well as information sharing (Konrad, 2007).

Shifting the Focus to Positive Interactions

Discussions in the literature have certainly contributed to increased appreciation of the importance of PHCP relationships with parents (Browning, 2002; Meyer et al., 2002) and of communication and humanizing interactions (Feudtner, 2007; Levetown and the American Academy of Pediatrics Committee on Bioethics, 2009; Meert et al., 2008). Yet we noted an enormous gap in research about how PHCPs can interact optimally with parents so they feel heard, respected, and cared for. Further, we discovered that the research base for caring for children with CCCs remains underdeveloped, particularly in acute care settings. Even literature from pediatric oncology and the neonatal intensive care unit (NICU)—settings in which many of these children are cared for—rarely elicited themes of optimizing interactions.

Even more astounding to us was the lack of acknowledgment that PHCPs may need to be explicitly taught not only about the principles of effective communication but also about how to interact effectively with patients and families. As health-care educators, we thought that PHCP education and training should extend beyond solely focusing on acquiring and generally applying a set of specific communication skills; providers also must become aware of how they themselves are affected by patients and families. In addition, we believed that there was a need for an understanding of how PHCPs' personal responses and other factors affect their interactions with patients and families and how they use (or do not use) communication skills. An interactional perspective was lacking—one that explores what patients and families expect and perceive that PHCPs bring into their relationships with them and, further, one that identifies what PHCPs expect from themselves and bring to such interactions in their pursuit of quality care (Papadatou, 2009). In other words, we noted a lack of understanding of what makes it possible for some, but not all, PHCPs to include both technical expertise and a generous sharing of their humanity. We understood:

> True service is not a relationship between an expert and a problem; it is far more genuine than that. It is a relationship between people who bring the full resources of their combined humanity to the table and share them generously. Service goes beyond expertise. Service is another way of life.
>
> (Remen, 2000, p. 198)

In this context, and to address the gap in our understanding about how to encourage and teach PHCPs to develop and maintain effective relationships, the long-term goal for our research was to provide meaningful guidance for optimizing the care of children with CCCs. For parents, such conditions are wrapped in uncertainty about causes, treatments, and outcomes; the shadow of death looms in the background. Parents often feel alone and vulnerable, and the nature of PHCPs' interactions with them is of critical importance. Our purpose was to develop an empirically grounded and theoretical conceptualization of what makes it possible for some PHCPs, more than others, to engage in excellent interactions with parents of children with serious illness. Thus, we designed the study that provides the foundation for this book.

Overview of the Foundational Project

Clearly, parents are affected not only by what PHCPs say but also by what they do and how they convey a sense of connection with, caring about, and compassion for individual parents and their ill child. We learned from previous research and clinical practice that improving our understanding about how PHCPs positively relate to parents across all types of interactions (e.g., technical, instructional, planned/spontaneous, or social) would contribute to optimizing pediatric palliative care for children and families.

It is our view that every encounter with another person involves an interaction, that is, an action that occurs because two or more people have an effect on one another. The idea of a two-way bidirectional effect, as opposed to a one-way causal effect, is essential in the concept of interaction. Interaction implies the activity of reciprocating or exchanging rather than simply giving (e.g., sharing rather than giving information). In our experience, communication is often perceived in health-care discussions as simply a means of transmitting information—imparting, sending, or giving information to others—often for the purpose of changing the behavior of others. As such, communication may be viewed as a means of control. Our study, however, focused on identifying and analyzing positive or human interactions rather than negative PHCP interactions with parents of children with CCCs.

The study of human interaction falls within the realm of natural inquiry, an approach to understanding the social world that involves collecting data from actual everyday life situations as they unfold. By engaging directly with research participants in field settings, naturalistic researchers draw on observations, interviews, and other sources of descriptive data, as well as their own subjective experiences, to create complex, holistic descriptions and interpretations of social phenomena that incorporate the human element (Tullis Owen, 2008). This approach contrasts with the perhaps more familiar quantitative approach in health care that attempts to separate the human element, employs laboratory or survey research, and focuses on measurement and analysis of causal relationships between variables that can be controlled. More simply put, quantitative research focuses on the trees, seeing them more distinctly by focusing on the trees' details, whereas qualitative research focuses on the forest to provide a broad perspective of the whole. Researchers in both traditions, however, use disciplined approaches as they seek answers to questions in health care, and both traditions are necessary when developing clinical care that has meaning for patients and their families. Quantitative researchers focus on counting specific aspects of health care, whereas qualitative researchers typically focus on what matters to individuals during their experience of health care.

Our study was guided by symbolic interactionism (SI), a term coined by sociologist Herbert Blumer (1969) that refers to a sociological theory developed by George Herbert Mead in the early part of the 20th century. This perspective relies on the symbolic meaning that people develop and depend upon in the process of social interaction in particular contexts. Social behaviors and cultural meanings are intertwined, and meanings arise from a number of elements, including one's perception of self (Blumer, 1969). SI addresses the subjective meanings that people impose on objects, events, and behaviors. Subjective meanings are given primacy because it is thought that people behave based on what they believe rather than just on what is objectively true. Thus, society is perceived as socially constructed through human interpretation. People interpret one another's behavior, and it is these interpretations that form the social bond.

Our focus on SI required a qualitative approach, one that allowed for exploration of PHCPs' and parents' own words and experiences as well as observations of their interactions. SI is at the heart of grounded theory, a naturalistic approach that aims to understand the underlying social process within a particular context (Charmaz, 2006). We chose a combined grounded theory/ethnographic approach to generate a detailed, contextually based conceptualization of the process involved in excellent PHCP–parent interactions. Furthermore, our prospective design allowed us to focus on interactions as they occurred, so we could uncover what parents and PHCPs perceived as helpful and rewarding in their interactions, as well as the contributing factors that made excellent interactions possible. Without doubt, we observed some negative interactions, but in those cases we concentrated on how the interactions affected the participants, how they differed from interactions that were fulfilling, and what participants would like to change in future interactions.

With ethics approval, we interviewed 34 parents of children with CCCs who were of a variety of ages and in any of three settings: Pediatric oncology and NICU in a children's hospital, and a free-standing children's hospice in Western Canada. We also interviewed 80 PHCPs who were primarily nurses ($N = 46$), physicians ($N = 19$), and social workers ($N = 5$), with chaplains, counselors, a child life specialist, a physiotherapist, an occupational therapist, and respiratory therapists accounting for the remaining 10 PHCPs. We also engaged in 88 ethnographic observations of PHCP–parent interactions. In addition, members of our team observed 18 of the 80 PHCPs who were interviewed (two of them twice for a total of 20 observations) while accompanying them for up to two hours during clinical activities. For each observation, team members wrote processual field notes documenting actual occurrences and investigator impressions of such aspects as nonverbal communication, responsiveness of parents and PHCPs to each other's cues, emotional atmosphere, potentially influencing factors, investigator impressions of reciprocity, and questions for follow-up during interviews. Finally, we conducted 51 general observations and conversations across the three settings to gain a greater understanding of each of these contexts.

Using QSR NVivo 10 (NVivo, 2014) to manage our data, we followed grounded theory procedures for analysis that were iterative from the start. PHCP and parent interviews were analyzed separately, initially by three team members experienced in qualitative research achieving consensus on the codes, their relationships, and the emerging conceptualization, and then with input from all other team members. Findings indicated that some PHCPs across disciplines demonstrated exemplary interactions. These providers engaged authentically and with intention in every encounter with parents, regardless of parents' characteristics or contributions to the interaction. Further, exemplary human-to-human exchanges were not simply the absence or the converse of negative or bad exchanges with parents. Rather, the model that we have articulated reflected something that has been inferred but not well described in the literature—that the components and specific facets of exemplary provider–parent interaction can be identified, described, and, ultimately, taught and learned.

Situating Our Study

When families come into the health-care system, they come for diagnosis/ treatment of a health condition. Their ultimate goal is to have the best possible outcome given the circumstance. Most PHCPs enter their profession because they want to help others. Current Westernized health-care systems have made great progress and have everyday success in the diagnosis and treatment of complex medical conditions. Yet we still see that patients and families are distressed with their experiences in the health-care system, many providers are experiencing burnout, and parents identify very few providers as excellent. Our goal is to help PHCPs learn how to practice in a way that both supports families and helps the providers feel that they are doing what they entered their profession to do. The focus of our study was on exemplary practice, and we would argue that the exemplary practices we describe in this book are the necessary prerequisites for optimal outcomes for patients and families—PHCPs cannot ensure well-being without these practices.

The Next Chapters

In the next 11 chapters, we will describe the overall model and its components, providing readers with an in-depth understanding of how to apply the model to their own practice. However, unlike other books, we will not offer separate sections or chapters about specific populations or diversity, for example, socially disadvantaged immigrant families or systemic racism. Rather, we will demonstrate how the model can be used in any situation, including those in which there may be challenges to optimal interaction because of differences among the participants, which highlights use of the model as one way to begin to address systemic racism and other isms in health care. We recognize that interactions are initiated when patients and families communicate with a PHCP but that not all patients and families are alike and not all patients and families are similar to all providers. A fundamental aspect of our model is that exemplary pediatric health-care providers (EPPs) pay attention to each patient/family member as an individual human being and strive to understand that person's needs and wants. Further, it is clear from the model that providers need to understand themselves and their own strengths and weaknesses so that they can continually self-monitor for potential biases and then take action as needed to correct such biases. In the end, the model is about how PHCPs engage with other human beings regardless of educational level, socio-demographic status, gender, race, and so on. When truly following the model, providers see differences not just as challenges to optimal interaction but also as opportunities to learn about another and for self-growth. Implications of the model are discussed in the final chapter.

Our conceptualization provides empirical evidence that EPP interaction is rooted in an encompassing *worldview* that results in specific *values* and a *commitment to authentic engagement* with and *empowerment* of parents. Their worldview is founded in the depth and breadth of providers' *knowledge*, persistent *curiosity, flexibility/open-mindedness*, and *self-awareness*. It is influenced by providers' *past experience, self-care*, and the *context* within which encounters occur. Central to EPP interaction while engaged in giving *direct care* and employing *connecting behaviors* is the process of *exquisitely attuning to particularities of the situation in the present moment*. This basic social process creates a *milieu of mattering*, a climate that allows for *positive outcomes* for both the parents and the providers. The conceptualization, represented metaphorically by a prairie windmill for purposes of knowledge translation, is discussed in Chapter 2.

References

American Association of Colleges of Nursing. (2018). *ELNEC curricula*. www.aacnnurs ing.org/ELNEC/About/ELNEC-Curricula

Baumeister, R. F., Bratslavsky, E., Finkenauer, C., & Vohs, K. D. (2001). Bad is stronger than good. *Review of General Psychology, 5*(4), 323–370. https://doi. org/10.1037/1089-2680.5.4.323

Blumer, H. (1969). *Symbolic interactionism: Perspective and method*. Prentice Hall.

Bonanno, G. A., Papa, A., Moskowitz, J. T., & Folkman, S. (2005). Resilience to loss in bereaved spouses, bereaved parents, and bereaved gay men. *Journal of Personality and Social Psychology, 88*(5), 827–483. https://doi.org/10.1037/0022-3514.88.5.827

Browning, D. (2002). To show our humanness—Relational and communicative competence in pediatric palliative care. *Bioethics Forum, 18*(3–4), 23–28. http://pdfs.seman ticscholar.org/c27b/fde0755cfec6ce7be8b639a61ed2015be835.pdf

Butler, A., Hall, H., Willetts, G., & Copnell, B. (2015). Parents' experiences of health care provider actions when their child dies: An integrative review of the literature. *Journal for Specialists in Pediatric Nursing, 20*(1), 5–20. https://doi.org/10.1111/ jspn.12097

Cadell, S., Hemsworth, D., Smit Quosai, T., Steele, R., Davies, E., Liben, S., Stratmann, L., & Siden, H. (2014). Posttraumatic growth in parents caring for a child with a life-limiting illness: A structural equation model. *American Journal of Orthopsychiatry, 84*(2), 123–133. https://doi.org/10.1037/h0099384

Charmaz, K. (2006). *Constructing grounded theory: A practical guide through qualitative analysis*. Sage.

Chou, W.-Y. S., Stokes, S. C., Citko, J., & Davies, B. (2008). Improving end-of-life care through community-based grassroots collaboration: Development of the Chinese-American coalition for compassionate care. *Journal of Palliative Care, 24*(1), 31–40. https://doi.org/10.1177/082585970802400105

Contro, N. A., Davies, B., Larson, J. M., & Sourkes, B. (2010). Away from home: Experiences of Mexican American families in pediatric palliative care. *Journal of Social Work in End-of-Life & Palliative Care, 6*(3–4), 185–204. https://doi.org/10.1080/15524256 .2010.529020

Contro, N. A., Larson, J., Scofield, S., Sourkes, B., & Cohen, H. J. (2002). Family perspectives on the quality of pediatric palliative care. *Archives of Pediatrics & Adolescent Medicine, 156*(1), 14–19. https://doi.org/0.1001/archpedi.156.1.14

Contro, N. A., Larson, J., Scofield, S., Sourkes, B., & Cohen, H. J. (2004). Hospital staff and family perspectives regarding quality of pediatric palliative care. *Pediatrics, 114*(5), 1248–1252. https://doi.org/10.1542/peds.2003-0857-L

Davies, B., Baird, J., & Gudmundsdottir, M. (2013). Moving family-centered care forward: Bereaved fathers' perspectives. *Journal of Hospice & Palliative Nursing, 15*, 163–170. https://doi.org/10.1097/NJH.0b013e3182765a2a

Davies, B., Collins, J., Steele, R., Cook, K., Distler, V., & Brenner, A. (2007). Parents' and children's perspectives of a children's hospice bereavement program. *Journal of Palliative Care, 23*(1), 14–23. https://doi.org/10.1177/082585970702300103

Davies, B., Contro, N., Larson, J., & Widger, K. (2010). Culturally-sensitive information-sharing in pediatric palliative care. *Pediatrics, 125*(4), e859–e865. https://doi.org/10.1542/peds.2009-0722

Davies, B., & Gudmundsdottir, M. (2006). *Fathers in pediatric end-of-life care* [Unpublished raw data]. School of Nursing and Health Professions, University of San Francisco.

Davies, B., Gudmundsdottir, M., Worden, B., Orloff, S., Sumner, L., & Brenner, P. (2004). "Living in the dragon's shadow": Fathers' experiences of a child's life-limiting illness. *Death Studies, 28*(2), 111–135. https://doi.org/10.1080/07481180490254501

Davies, B., Larson, J., Contro, N., & Cabrera, B. (2011). Perceptions of discrimination among Mexican American families of seriously ill children. *Journal of Palliative Medicine, 14*(1), 71–76. https://doi.org/10.1089/jpm.2010.0315

Feudtner, C. (2007). Collaborative communication in pediatric palliative care: A foundation for problem-solving and decision-making. *Pediatric Clinics of North America, 54*(5), 583–607. https://doi.org/10.1016/j.pcl.2007.07.008

Feudtner, C., Christakis, D. A., & Connell, F. A. (2000). Pediatric deaths attributable to complex chronic conditions: A population-based study of Washington state. *Pediatrics, 106*, 205–209. https://pediatrics.aappublications.org/content/pediatrics/106/Supplement_1/205.full.pdf

Garwick, A. W., Kohrman, C., Wolman, C., & Blume, R. W. (1998). Families' recommendations for improving services for children with chronic conditions. *Archives of Pediatrics and Adolescent Medicine, 152*(5), 440–448. https://doi.org/10.1001/archpedi.152.5.440

Heller, K. S., & Solomon, M. Z. (2005). Continuity of care and caring: What matters to parents of children with life-threatening conditions. *Journal of Pediatric Nursing, 20*(5), 335–346. https://doi.org/10.1016/j.pedn.2005.03.005

Janzen, L., Cadell, S., & Westhues, A. (2003–2004). From death notification through the funeral: Bereaved parents' experiences and their advice to professionals. *Omega—Journal of Death and Dying, 48*(2), 149–164. https://doi.org/10.2190/6XUW-4PYD-H88Q-RQ08

Kolarik, R. C., Walker, G., & Arnold, R. M. (2006). Pediatric resident education in palliative care: A needs assessment. *Pediatrics, 117*(6), 1949–1954. https://doi.org/10.1542/peds.2005-1111

Konrad, S. C. (2007). What parents of seriously ill children value: Parent-to-parent connection and mentorship. *Omega—Journal of Death and Dying, 55*(2), 117–130. https://doi.org/10.2190/OM.55.2.b

Levetown, M. and the American Academy of Pediatrics Committee on Bioethics. (2009). Communicating with children and families: From everyday interactions to skill in conveying distressing information. *Pediatrics, 121*(5), e1441–e1460. https://doi.org/10.1542/peds.2008-0565

Macdonald, M. E., Liben, S., Carnevale, F. A., Rennick, J. E., Wolf, S. L., Meloche, D., & Cohen, S. R. (2005). Parental perspectives on hospital staff members' acts of kindness and commemoration after a child's death. *Pediatrics, 116*(4), 884–890. https://doi.org/10.1542/peds.2004-1980

Meert, K. L., Eggly, S., Pollack, M., Anand, K. J. S., Zimmerman, J., Carcillo, J., & Nicholson, C. (2008). Parents' perspectives on physician-parent communication near the time of a child's death in the pediatric intensive care unit. *Pediatric Critical Care Medicine, 9*, 2–7. https://doi.org/10.1097/01.PCC.0000298644.13882.88

Melin-Johansson, C., Axelsson, I., Grundberg, M. J., & Hallqvist, F. (2014). When a child dies: Parents' experiences of palliative care—An integrative literature review. *Journal of Pediatric Nursing, 29*(6), 660–669. https://doi.org/10.1016/j.pedn.2014.06.009

Meyer, E. C., Burns, J. P., Griffith, J. L., & Truog, R. D. (2002). Parental perspectives on end-of-life care in the pediatric intensive care unit. *Critical Care Medicine, 30*(1), 226–231.

Munet-Vilaro, F. (2004). Delivery of culturally competent care to children with cancer and their families—The Latino experience. *Journal of Pediatric Oncology Nursing, 21*(3), 155–159. https://doi.org/10.1177/1043454204264405

National Hospice and Palliative Care Organization. (2018). *Education.* www.nhpco.org/education

NVivo (Version 10). (2014). *Computer software.* QSR International Pty Ltd. www.qsrinternational.com/nvivo/home

Papadatou, D. (2009). *In the face of death: Professionals who care for the dying and the bereaved.* Springer.

Rehm, R. S. (1999). Religious faith in Mexican-Americans dealing with chronic childhood illness. *Image: Journal of Nursing Scholarship, 3*(1), 33–38. https://doi.org/10.1111/j.1547-5069.1999.tb00417.x

Remen, R. N. (2000). *My grandfather's blessings: Stories of strength, refuge, and belonging.* Riverhead Books.

Steele, R., & Davies, B. (2006). Impact on parents when a child has a progressive, life-threatening illness. *International Journal of Palliative Nursing, 12*(12), 576–585. https://doi.org/10.12968/ijpn.2006.12.12.22544

Sternberg, E. M. (2001). *The balance within: The science connecting health and emotions.* W. H. Freeman.

Stevenson, M., Achille, M., & Lugasi, T. (2013). Pediatric palliative care in Canada and the United States: A qualitative metasummary of the needs of patients and families. *Journal of Palliative Medicine, 16*(5), 566–577. https://doi.org/10.1089/jpm.2011.0076

Surkan, P. J., Kreicbergs, U., Valdimarsdottir, U., Nyberg, U., Onelov, E., Dickman, P. W., & Steineck, G. (2006). Perceptions of inadequate health care and feelings of guilt in parents after the death of a child to a malignancy: A population-based long-term follow-up. *Journal of Palliative Medicine, 9*(2), 317–331. https://doi.org/10.1089/jpm.2006.9.317

Tullis Owen, J. A. (2008). Naturalistic inquiry. In L. M. Given (Ed.), *The Sage encyclopedia of qualitative research methods* (Vol. 1, pp. 547–550). Sage.

van der Kolk, B. (2015). *The body keeps the score: Mind, brain and body in the transformation of trauma.* Penguin.

Woodgate, R. L. (2006). Living in a world without closure: Reality for parents who have experienced the death of a child. *Journal of Palliative Care, 22*(2), 75–82. https://doi.org/10.1177/082585970602200203

Xafis, V., Wilkinson, D., & Sullivan, J. (2015). What information do parents need when facing end-of-life decisions for their child? A meta-synthesis of parental feedback. *BMC Palliative Care, 14*(19), 1–11. https://doi.org/10.1186/s12904-015-0024-0

2 Metaphor and Overview of Model of Exemplary Interaction

The metaphor shows the whole of interaction, the movement back and forth of the many facets that are important. It captures the mystery of interaction, of the connection that really makes things happen. It's fun to play with because it really makes you think in a different way about excellence in interaction.

Metaphors

Human beings understand that when they build bridges between people, they are talking about connections that are not concrete structures. They know that when a captain calls for all hands on deck, he wants more than just hands. Metaphor is at the center of language and enables humans to make creative sense of what is around them. Since the time of Plato, metaphors have been a common means of expressing an understanding of complex concepts (Jensen, 2006). The word itself derives from the Latin metaphora, where "phor" is to carry over or to transfer and "meta" refers to meaning. Metaphors provide access to everyday practices and invite people into worlds that they might not have seen otherwise. By connecting information about one familiar concept to another familiar concept, the comparison between the two concepts can suggest another way of looking at one's everyday life, thus making it possible to uncover both individual and collective patterns of thought and action or, at least, to grasp inklings of possibilities for new perspectives (Schmitt, 2005). Metaphors can stimulate imagination, arouse feeling, help people to grasp these new meanings, and prompt them to action and change. In short, metaphors are excellent tools to help simplify complex concepts.

Metaphors are also one avenue for illuminating the meanings of research findings because they help researchers to describe complex concepts in a way that enables others to grasp the dimensions of a concept (Greene, 1994). They provide structure to data and aid understanding of a familiar process in a new light. In the research study that is the foundation for this book, we (the authors) used metaphor for this purpose. Our project was one not of metaphorical analysis (i.e., the analysis of metaphors described by participants) but of creating a metaphor for the purpose of clarifying and presenting our findings in a useful way.

The use of metaphor enables the examination of the phenomena under study from a unique and creative perspective and is particularly useful when

DOI: 10.4324/9780429352393-2

researchers are neck deep in data and cannot see the forest for the trees. At such times, it can be hard to get a wide-enough angle on the research question to draw broad inferences, and a metaphor allows researchers to find associations quickly through the power of unconscious processing (Lakoff & Johnson, 2003). Our project, as with many qualitative research projects, yielded a multitude of pieces of information that contained complex meaningful structures. Knowing that visual representation of the emerging concepts and their connections is an intrinsic and essential step in grounded theory analysis, we drew multiple diagrams and relational maps to help us see the meaning in our data in more ways than just words alone (Verdinelli & Scagnoli, 2013). Such configurations often result in the identification of a metaphor that aids not only in further analysis but also in providing access to and understanding of the situation under study.

Importantly, the use of metaphor should not be seen as forced simplification; metaphors only become useful if they make interpretation possible, that is, if knowledge users can make a connection between the concepts, the events, thoughts, and actions that take place in the real world (Schmitt, 2005). We found that a windmill metaphor helped us make sense of our research findings. This metaphor allowed us to provide a scheme that bundled together the fullness of details, making them clearer and more manageable, and became a vital part of being able to make sense of things. Equally important, our windmill drawing enabled us to share our findings with study participants and nonparticipants alike in ways that made sense to their experiences of interactions with patients, families, colleagues, and others.

Developing Our Windmill Metaphor

As we analyzed the ever-increasing mounds of data, we began to identify the many aspects of EPP–parent interaction. We eventually discovered that EPPs who were perceived as *exquisite* in connecting with others enacted these aspects both all at once and nearly all of the time, depending on factors such as their internal and external resources and parents' ability to engage. We wondered how to best represent these all-at-once behaviors so they were seen as one, as an inseparable whole when in action. Given our background in pediatrics, a child's pinwheel came to mind because when blown the individual petals disappear as they spin in unison to create one whirling sphere. But a pinwheel's construction was far too simple to adequately represent the behaviors and the other factors that we discovered came into play during EPP–parent interaction. Having grown up surrounded by the Canadian prairies, Betty was familiar with the sight of windmills stationed across the extended patchwork of fields, spinning in the wind to pump water for human, animal, and agricultural survival. A prairie water-pumping windmill seemed a good fit to metaphorically represent our important observation and the overall complexity of EPP–parent interactions.

As we continued with our analysis, it became clear that the windmill was the perfect metaphor because it helped us depict how the various components of exemplary interaction were interrelated and led to optimal outcomes.

Participants in our presentations told us that the metaphor resonated with them emotionally rather than just intellectually. Because of the windmill metaphor, they identified a deeper understanding of the essence of exemplary interaction and saw opportunities for change in practice, education, and administration.

How a Water-Pumping Windmill Works

The more we considered the possibility of a windmill as our metaphor, the more we wanted to ensure that we were knowledgeable about water-pumping windmills so we could be clear on how the windmill illuminated our findings (see Figure 2.1). We also needed to be able to answer questions that arose when we presented our research findings to our study participants and other audiences because we discovered that some people, like Betty's husband who grew up in the suburbs of Chicago, did not know how a windmill worked. It was fascinating to learn that windmills represent one of the key pieces of technology that enabled our ancestors to transform the power of the wind into a physical force that could be used for numerous purposes. Though it is uncertain which civilization can lay claim to being the first to use the wind as a mechanical power source on land, when this event actually occurred, or what its impetus may have been, historians have documented that windmills have been in operation for at least 1,000 years.

Despite their popularity being dramatically reduced after the arrival of steam- and electricity-powered machines in the 19th and 20th centuries, windmills were, and still are today, actively used all around the world. In the North American west, settlement of the dry grasslands and prairies was almost impossible before the development of the first windmill by Halliday in 1854 (Baker, 1985). Thereafter, windmills pumped underground water to the surface, supplied the needs of farmers and ranchers, and became the most prominent feature of the Western landscape (Baker, 1985). Today's wind-electric turbines may be ubiquitous, but they are unable to portray the complexity of human interaction that the classic windmill provides.

The workings of a water-pumping windmill are complicated to non-engineers like the three of us. We read several detailed descriptions of the construction and mechanics of windmills, but for our metaphorical purposes, we hope that a simple description will suffice. We trust that readers who are more mechanically inclined will tolerate (or forgive) our simplistic interpretation. Most traditional water-pumping windmills consist of three main parts: The windwheel comprises (1) the blades or sails with their stabilizing bands, the hub and rudder assembly, the gearing assembly, and the shaft, (2) the tower, and (3) the pumping mechanism. Each piece of the windmill, like a three-legged stool, is useless without the other. Each part is engineered with a specific purpose to ensure efficient and long-lasting operation in the field.

Water-pumping windmills feature a number of blades or sails that turn in the wind. A rudder sits behind the sail mechanism and turns the sails in the direction of the wind to maximize the sails' efficiency. The sails are

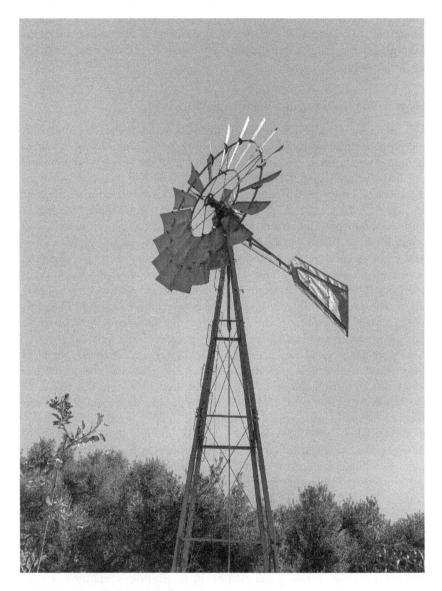

Figure 2.1 Photograph of a Water-Pumping Windmill

rigidly mounted at an angle to the wind. As the wind passes through the opening between the sails, it is compressed on the face of the sail. As it exits the windwheel, an area of low pressure is created behind the sail. It is this difference in pressure that applies a force against the sail, causing it to rotate. A gearbox and crankshaft convert this rotary motion into reciprocating strokes carried downward through a rod or shaft to the pump cylinder below, thus bringing up water from the ground.

Overall Fit Between Windmills and Exemplary Interaction

As we learned about windmills, we came to appreciate even more ways in which they represent our conceptualization of EPP–parent interaction. For example, windmills have been in use for over a millennium because they have enduring utility. They are actually simple devices, a modern form of historic technology, that remain useful today on the plains of not only North America but also Australia, New Zealand, Namibia, and, more recently, China. Exemplary interaction between persons also has enduring utility and is relevant across all areas of health care, within all cultures, and among all peoples.

Windmills were developed for delivering water for human sustenance in areas where the only source of water was underground; without the windmill, human life on the prairies would not have survived. Our windmill represents the nature of interaction that is necessary for optimal outcomes in health-care delivery; without human-to-human interaction, we believe that optimal outcomes in health-care settings are threatened. The farmers and ranchers who use windmills see them as reliable, lasting more than 70 years with regular maintenance. Similarly, parents perceive EPPs as trustworthy and reliable, providing memories of encounters that continue to offer parents comfort for years following their child's illness and/or death. Further, EPPs' colleagues also see them as trustworthy and reliable team members who contribute to optimal team functioning.

Although many have attempted to improve the current windmill design, it still stands unchallenged as the most practical design yet produced. Gillis (2015), a windmill historian, pointed out that the design has been so well refined that small changes, even to the surface of the sail, result in a reduction of pumping ability. Similarly, we believe that our model of EPP–parent interaction provides a most practical design for humanizing health care and that omitting any single component results in less than optimal outcomes for both parents and providers.

Finally, besides their practical utility, windmills hold a special place in many aspects of life—in poetry, literature, film imagery, architecture, language, even mini-golf courses (Lombardo, 2003)—so too with our model. Although the model is derived from and applies to PHCPs, it represents exemplary interactions that were evident across disciplines, age groups, and settings.

Our Windmill Metaphor of Exemplary Pediatric Provider Interaction

It is important to remember that all components and facets of the windmill must work together dynamically for optimal functioning, but in this section we will discuss each aspect of the windmill sequentially. As you move forward in the book, you will notice that some aspects of the model are discussed in more than one chapter. This overlap reflects the interconnectedness of the model components and the consequences of our attempt to discuss a holistic model in discrete chapters.

The presentation format in this section provides an overview of each component of the windmill and its relevance to interactions. Our intention is that this description will allow you to see the whole before we begin to discuss each component in depth.

Families (Wind)

By catching the wind, just like the sails on a sailboat, the blades on a windmill turn the windwheel. Without the wind, there is no movement. Similarly, in our model, without families there is no interaction between parents and PHCPs. How the wind blows is beyond human control—and so were the families that PHCPs served. Some families presented with a calm demeanor, had higher levels of functioning, were open and adaptable, and were like a gentle breeze. Other families were characterized by an unsettled manner, were less open to change, had difficulty expressing themselves, were reluctant to engage with others, and presented as a strong wind. Regardless of the nature of a family's way of being in the world, EPPs consistently sought ways of engaging with each family member to achieve the best possible outcome for that particular family. The crucial components and specific facets of the conceptualization of EPP interaction with parents are outlined in Table 2.1, and the relationships between and among these components, using the windmill metaphor, are illustrated in Figure 2.2.

Worldview and Values (Rudder)

Not always clearly visible behind the windwheel (the blades) of a windmill, nor appreciated for its central role in optimizing the windmill's function, the windmill rudder turns the windwheel in the direction of the wind so that the blades can optimally capture the wind's energy. Similarly, the *worldview* and *values* of EPPs who excelled at interaction turned the blades in the direction of the patient and family so as to optimally engage with them.

Commitment to Authentic Engagement (Hub)

The hub, located at the center of the windwheel, is the central point where all the moving parts come together. It is the connecting point for the windwheel and the rudder, for the gearbox and the central shaft—all of which are integral to the viability of the windmill. For EPPs, their hub was a *commitment to authentic engagement*. It was the point where their *worldview* and *values* connected with an awareness of their direct contribution, both as professionals and as persons, to the situation. Finally, the hub reflected their determination to know patients and families as people, not just as patients or parents, and to collaborate with them as partners in care.

Attuning (Blades)

The blades are central to how a windmill functions. The blades catch the wind and respond to it by spinning faster or slower depending on the wind's

Table 2.1 Components and Specific Facets of Exemplary Pediatric Health Care Provider/Parent Interaction

Components	Specific Facets of Each Component
Worldview and Values	• Fundamental orientation to how one exists in the world.
	• Expansive perspective, seeing the world as a whole.
	• Encompassing life's many processes and paradoxes, privileges and inequities.
	• Trusting in life, in other people, in the potential of humankind, and in making meaning of their work.
	• Respecting the worth of all persons.
	• Valuing diversity.
	• Valuing social justice, providing equitable care to all.
	• Engaging in family-centered care.
	• Maintaining personal and professional integrity.
Commitment to Authentic Engagement	• Recognizing the interconnectivity and complexity of human relationships.
	• Striving to know parents as people.
	• Making time for engagement with parents.
Core Social Process of Attuning	• Engaging in all six facets at the same time.
	• Orienting.
	• Seeking parents' perspectives.
	• Discerning.
	• Shaping.
	• Checking.
	• Reflecting.
Direct Care Activities—Doing-For	• Administering treatments, carrying out procedures.
	• Attending to physical care.
	• Managing technology.
	• Seeking consultation from other professionals.
	• Referring to other services.
Direct Care Activities—Empowering	• Navigating.
	• Supporting.
	• Sharing information.
	• Teaching.
Connecting Behaviors	• Empathizing.
	• Showing kindness.
	• Suspending judgment.
	• Building and maintaining trust.
	• Listening.
	• Pacing the message.
	• Maintaining hope.
	• Staying positive.
Personal Influencing Factors	• Knowledge.
	• Self-awareness.
	• Flexibility/Open-mindedness.
	• Curiosity.
	• Self-care.
	• Past experience.

Components	Specific Facets of Each Component
Relationship	• Establishing relationship. • Developing relationship. • Ending relationship. • Professional relationship vs. friendship. • Maintaining boundaries. • Challenges to maintaining boundaries.
Setting and Team Contextual Factors: Immediate Work Environment	• Priority of care in setting. • Fit with setting. • Contributing to optimal teamwork. • Challenges in teamwork.
Institutional and Societal Contextual Factors: Broader Environment	• Serving a pediatric population. • Relative richness of pediatric funding and resources. • Impact of policies and procedures on delivery of pediatric care. • Quality of leadership at institutional and setting levels. • Corporatization of health care. • Working in a technological world. • Societal attitudes towards death.
Output: Milieu of Mattering	• Sense of belonging, mattering to each other. • Concerns matter to each other. • United, committed to common interest. • Respected, valued; human dignity intact. • Openness, expressiveness. • Making a difference.

force. Similarly, central to exemplary interaction was how EPPs responded to parents according to individual situations and what mattered most to a parent at the time. This process, *attuning to the particularities of the situation in the moment*, involved six interrelated and intertwined facets (blades) of interaction: *Orienting, seeking parents' perspectives, discerning, sharing, checking,* and *reflecting.* A defining characteristic of exemplary interaction was that EPPs conscientiously engaged in each facet while simultaneously enacting all facets in a recurrent and iterative manner.

Direct Care Activities (Inner Stabilizing Band)

Stabilizing bands support and protect a windmill's blades from bending, breaking, or falling apart. The bands also provide strength to hold the wind-wheel together in strong winds when the centrifugal forces can be great. If the blades are not reinforced and properly balanced, the whole assembly may wobble or even collapse. In PHCP interaction, the inner stabilizing band represents the direct care activities that all PHCPs are obligated to carry out as part of their professional role. It is through such activities that provider–patient encounters most often occurred. Direct care activities were

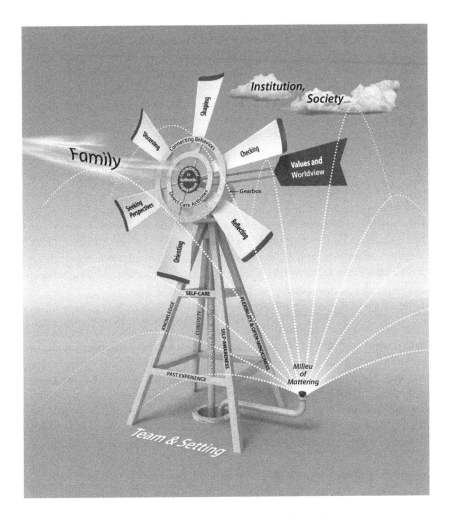

Figure 2.2 Model of EPP–Parent Interaction: A Windmill Metaphor

of two types: *Doing-for* and *empowering*. The overall goal of doing-for was to do for patients/families what they could not do for themselves. Doing-for activities were *administering treatments* or *carrying out procedures, attending to physical care, managing technology, seeking consultation*, and *referring*. Empowering patients and family members was a top priority for EPPs. They strove to enable patients and family members to do what they wanted and needed to do rather than taking over and doing it for them. The four empowering activities were *navigating, sharing information, supporting*, and *teaching*. Though some direct care activities were more prevalent in some disciplines, EPPs across disciplines engaged in all types of direct care activities to some degree.

Connecting Behaviors (Outer Stabilizing Band)

The outer stabilizing band represents the relational behaviors that were inherent in all exemplary encounters and that arose from EPPs' commitment to authentic engagement in interaction with parents and family members. The connecting behaviors were *building and maintaining trust, listening, empathizing, pacing, focusing on positive, suspending judgment, showing kindness,* and *maintaining hope.* These behaviors permeated every aspect of the encounter. They were skills that were necessary but not sufficient by themselves for PHCPs to optimally attune to the needs and concerns of patients and family members.

Personal Influencing Factors (Legs and Struts)

The legs and struts comprise the supporting framework for a windmill. The legs provide strong and secure grounding, while the struts reinforce and brace the legs. Likewise, four characteristics (*knowledge, self-awareness, flexibility/open-mindedness,* and *curiosity*) and two struts (*past experience* and *self-care*) worked together in providing a solid foundation for exemplary interaction.

EPP–Parent Relationship (Shaft)

Also attached to a windmill's hub, along with the rudder and the blades, is the gearbox and the rod or shaft. In the gearbox, the wind's energy is converted into mechanical energy that rotates a central vertical shaft, creating motion that is then used to pump water out of the ground. In our model, the energy generated by the process of *attuning* while engaged in *direct care activities* and *connecting behaviors* was converted into a mutually respectful, dialogical, and meaningful EPP–parent *relationship* (the shaft) that characterized exemplary interaction and maintained professional and personal *boundaries.*

Contextual Influencing Factors (Ground and Climate)

Unlike the personal influencing factors, the contextual factors were external to the PHCPs. One group of factors (ground)—*team* and *setting*—was particular to the immediate work environment. In order to provide optimal stability, windmills are built upon solid ground, not sandy, rocky, or cracked earth. Similarly, exemplary interaction was grounded within an EPP's health-care team in the particular setting. The level of team functioning and leadership, as well as a setting's particular history, the focus of care provided in that setting, and its unit culture, all contributed to the *milieu of mattering* that EPPs created through interaction. When the team and/or setting were not optimal, EPPs sometimes struggled to achieve exemplary interaction, but they still found a way to engage authentically.

The second group of factors—*institution* and *society*—encompassed two aspects of the broader environment (climate). Located on open land, windmills are subject to the elements of nature—for example, blazing sunshine, sudden hailstorms, or freezing blizzards—that affect not only the windmill but also the ground upon which it sits. Similarly, PHCP interaction was influenced by the institutional setting, including leadership at the unit and institutional levels, and the broader society in which PHCPs work. EPPs were well aware of these factors and worked creatively to deal with and remove the challenges where possible; despite challenges, they still managed to demonstrate exemplary interaction.

Output (Water)

An effective prairie windmill pumps life-giving water out of the ground. Similarly, as a result of exemplary interactions, EPPs' created a *milieu of mattering* (output) in which both parents and EPPs felt that they and their concerns mattered to each other and that they were not alone when facing the challenges of caring for children with CCCs. Parents felt that they and those who mattered most to them—their children—were treated with respect and with their human dignity intact. EPPs felt similarly respected and valued by parents. Both EPPs and parents felt that they were making a difference in the lives of one another. Further, while working within their team to make a difference in the lives of families, EPPs engaged in exemplary interactions with their colleagues and contributed to team members feeling that they belonged and mattered to each other.

The windmill metaphor is useful in explaining the seemingly simple but complex process of exemplary interaction because each component of the model can be separately described, but it also illustrates how the many facets of interaction occur simultaneously. Each component is essential but insufficient in and of itself to achieve the exemplary interaction that EPPs showed. Parents and peers alike recognized EPPs as being the best at what they do. PHCPs could be adept at carrying out one or more of the components and be seen as providing good care, but it was only when PHCPs carried out all facets that they were considered to be EPPs. Our intent is certainly not to imply that some PHCPs are doing it all wrong and others are doing it all right. Rather, as one of our participants articulated, we desire to make good care even better. We offer our model as a way of enhancing interaction with the intent of preventing, or at least alleviating, the negative outcomes that arise from less than optimal encounters.

Using the Windmill Metaphor for Knowledge Translation

A large gulf remains between what clinicians know and what they practice. Research into health and health care has achieved substantial advancement in knowledge and improvements in care through its focus on interventions, treatment, and cure. And yet, many researchers, educators, and clinicians frequently lament the lack of success in putting research findings into practice. In many cases, the traditional ways of disseminating knowledge are not sufficient.

Generally, it is expected that the purpose of research is to produce formal generalizations that can then be used by practitioners to guide their own practice in their own particular situations. Indeed, arguments in many health-care proposals reflect the belief that research leads to knowledge that leads to improved practice. But clinicians, when presented with this new knowledge and pressure to change as a result of it, may sense an underlying message that what they are doing is somehow deficient and must be abandoned. This sense of criticism is threatening to anyone, especially to clinicians who are focused on doing all they can to care for their patients in the best possible way and to educators who diligently teach health-care professionals (HCPs). Perhaps because health-care education has become so information-oriented, there is a deeply embedded expectation that knowledge alone could make HCPs adopt changes if researchers only provided the information gleaned from their research studies. But just as HCPs learned long ago that simply giving out information to the public about the effects of smoking or obesity does not motivate many individuals to stop smoking or to lose weight, researchers must find different ways of translating research findings if they are serious about facilitating changes in practice.

The Canadian Institutes of Health Research (2012) identified that when there are potential knowledge-user audiences beyond the research community, strategies for knowledge translation should be more intensive and emphasize nonacademic modes of communication; the language of publication should be adapted to the target audiences and presented in alternative formats. Straus et al. (2011) concurred and noted that to make knowledge useful for application in health-care settings, researchers must present findings in ways that they can be easily understood and capture the attention of the intended users of the knowledge. The windmill metaphor meets these recommendations. Clinicians and educators, as well as parents, patients, and other family members, have told us that the metaphor *speaks* to them so that the model *makes sense*. If we as researchers are serious about the well-being of practitioners and teachers, then we must present our findings in such a way that they touch or capture the personal experiences of practitioners and teachers so they can find personal meaning in the new knowledge. Yet finding new ways of disseminating knowledge can be constrained by existing publication requirements.

We submitted a paper to describe the preliminary overall findings from our study and included a windmill diagram to illustrate the various components of our conceptual model and the relationships between and among the components. However, the final diagram required by the journal editor prior to publishing our paper (see Davies et al., 2017) ended up comprising the lines, circles, and boxes joined by arrows typical of the traditional type of diagram found in many papers that report qualitative research findings. Yet when we showed that diagram along with our windmill diagram (see Figure 2.2) to workshop and conference participants, we received immediate feedback that the windmill captured participants' attention, aroused their interest, and made the whole of interactions much easier to understand. In fact, audience members told us that the windmill diagram motivated them to want to learn more about our model because they could see how it works and how it fits with their own experiences:

The windmill is really insightful, much more creative, dynamic, and transformational. I think what's brilliant to me about this model is that there are so many elements and to try to figure out which ones are connected at which level or layer and how they all work, the wholeness of it—I think it's really wonderful.

Using metaphors to translate research results is less formal or structured than the usual academic ways in which researchers present their findings; it is more than simply being offered some new information. Through comparison, the metaphor allows others to experience and understand one thing in terms of another; the facts become interpretable, or make sense, in regard to their place within the metaphoric structure (Richardson, 2003). Moreover, effective change most often occurs incrementally, so if the imagination or the emotion of an audience can be tapped, then a more evolutionary change may result and, in the long run, be more effective in putting new knowledge into practice. Our goal with this book is to invite you, the reader, into our metaphor so you can learn how, or teach someone else how, to achieve exemplary interaction. We begin in Chapter 3 by discussing *worldview*, *values*, and *authentic engagement*.

References

Baker, T. L. (1985). *A field guide to American windmills*. University of Oklahoma Press.

Canadian Institutes of Health Research. (2012). *Guide to knowledge translation planning at CIHR: Integrated and end-of-grant approaches*. https://cihr-irsc.gc.ca/e/documents/kt_lm_ktplan-en.pdf

Davies, B., Steele, R., Krueger, G., Albersheim, S., Baird, J., Bifirie, M., Cadell, S., Doane, S., Garga, D., Siden, H., Strahlendorf, C., & Zhou, Y. (2017). Best practices in provider/parent interaction. *Qualitative Health Research*, *27*(3), 406–420. https://doi.org/0.1177/1049732316664712

Gillis, C. C. (2015). *Still turning: A history of aermotor windmills*. A&M University Press.

Greene, M. (1994). Epistemology and educational research: The influence of recent approaches to knowledge. *Review of Research in Education*, *20*, 423–464. www.jstor.org/stable/1167390

Jensen, D. F. N. (2006). Metaphors as a bridge to understanding educational and social contexts. *International Journal of Qualitative Methods*, *5*(1), 36–54. https://journals.sagepub.com/doi/pdf/10.1177/160940690600500104

Lakoff, G., & Johnson, M. (2003). *Metaphors we live by*. University of Chicago Press. http://shu.bg/tadmin/upload/storage/161.pdf

Lombardo, D. (2003). *Windmills of New England: Their genius, madness, history and future*. On Cape Publications.

Richardson, L. (2003). Writing: A method of inquiry. In N. K. Denzin & V. S. Lincoln (Eds.), *Collecting and interpreting qualitative materials* (2nd ed., pp. 499–541). Sage.

Schmitt, R. (2005). Systematic metaphor analysis as a method of qualitative research. *The Qualitative Report*, *10*(2), 358–394. https://nsuworks.nova.edu/cgi/viewcontent.cgi?article=1854&context=tqr

Straus, S. E., Tetroe, J. M., & Graham, I. D. (2011). Knowledge translation is the use of knowledge in health care decision making. *Journal of Clinical Epidemiology*, *64*(1), 6–10. https://doi.org/10.1016/j.jclinepi.2009.08.016

Verdinelli, S., & Scagnoli, N. I. (2013). Data display in qualitative research. *International Journal of Qualitative Methods*, *12*, 359–381. https://journals.sagepub.com/doi/pdf/10.1177/160940691301200117

3 Worldview, Values, and Commitment to Authentic Engagement

If I think of what grounds me in my work, it's my worldview. My worldview about the human condition is believing in the potential of others and knowing that there will always be life and death, distress and joy—both are part of what life is and that's not going to change. While I'm here I'll do the best I can; it's like accepting the mystery. It's a really strong foundation of trust in a process that is constantly unfolding. It's the trust we have in one another—the essence of living—that's how I can keep doing the work that I do.

Worldview/Values

As we (authors) write this chapter, the news of today's world seems filled with stories of loss and human suffering—from fires, droughts, floods, hurricanes, and volcanoes, to photos of children separated from their families at the US border, to stories of starving children due to war and political upheaval. Reports of political corruption abound as do personal accounts about how many education and health-care systems have become increasingly bureaucratic, cold, and impersonal. It is easy to wonder if, in today's world, it is harder to be human than it used to be. Perhaps that is one reason why the parents of children with life-threatening conditions told us how much it meant to them when PHCPs treated them as human beings. Maybe it is why parents also said that PHCPs who do so—the excellent or exemplary ones—were so few in number. The research question for our study then became, "What makes it possible for those health-care providers to be seen as excellent or exemplary?" And we found that our answers started with their worldview.

A person's worldview is the fundamental orientation to how they exist in the world; it creates or is responsible for the perceptual filters through which each person views the world. Consequently, people's lives and actions then seek to express their worldview. In our model, EPPs' worldview and the resulting values are represented by the rudder of the windmill. The rudder is not always clearly visible behind the blades of a windmill, nor is it often appreciated for its central role in optimizing the windmill's function. The rudder moves the windwheel in the direction of the wind to catch it in the most effective way. In turn, this motion is responsible for

DOI: 10.4324/9780429352393-3

making the pump work. Similarly, EPPs' worldview and values turn their attention in the direction of the parents so they can catch whatever the parent is offering and, thus, optimally respond to and engage with parents. Regardless of the nature of any particular encounter with parents—whether it is meeting for the first time, explaining the child's diagnosis, completing a procedure for the child, teaching parents about the child's care, or simply passing one another in the hallway—EPPs' worldview and values guide every interaction.

Though worldviews can be radically different from one another, EPPs have in common a worldview that incorporates an expansive perspective on the human condition and all its complexities, diversities, and ambiguities. They see the world as a whole, incorporating life's many processes and paradoxes, privileges and inequities. Their worldview encompasses the good and the bad, the bright and the dark, the happy and the sad, the successes and the failures of people, situations, and environments. EPPs need not just kindness but also the courage to face the dark side of life. They perceive these many facets of the human condition as interconnected, interdependent, multifunctional, emotional, rational, and spiritual, continuously affecting and shaping one another. EPPs do not believe that each individual is alone in the world as an independent, autonomous being; rather, they see that all people are connected to and affected by others and, as a result, everybody counts. They understand and appreciate the commonality among all people because we *are all united in attachment, loss, love, and grief. We are all part of the global tribe who share these things. It's about community and being there for one another and that's what keeps us going as a society.* Some EPPs' worldview, particularly for chaplains, includes a religious or spiritual aspect (either in affiliation or practice), but all EPPs demonstrate a trust in life, in other people, in the potential of humankind, and in making meaning of their work.

Despite holding a large and inclusive worldview, EPPs are not simply idealists. They are aware of the interdependent, systemic reach of their own actions—the ripple effects of words, decisions, and behaviors. They understand themselves to be working on behalf of the whole of life, making the world a better place by making a positive difference in the lives of seriously ill children and their parents, by making the parents' traumatic experience as good as a bad experience can be. They treat every interaction as an opportunity to learn and connect, rather than to perform and do. As a result, parents feel accepted as valued members of the team.

Embedded in EPPs' encompassing worldview is a deep respect for parents, regardless of age, culture, gender, intelligence, status, or any other difference between themselves and parents. Their assumption is that each parent has innate worth, value, and dignity and should be treated with interest, warmth, patience, civility, compassion, and decency. They highly regard parents' individual experiences and give parents the benefit of the doubt by assuming that parents are doing the best they can to cope with all that comes with having a seriously ill child. Seeing parents as fellow human beings enables EPPs to understand much about the complexity of and ambiguity within and outside of themselves and to see how that also is the case for parents. They can imagine the parent's situation and then see themselves in it; they can feel compassion:

> How can we look at dying directly as a way to make it as meaningful, as reconciling, as beautiful a remembrance as possible? Because the actual act of dying is awful, so how do we hear and interpret what would be important for that family during the event?

EPPs are identifiable because of how their worldview is demonstrated in their respectful approach to parents. Their deep regard for the human condition moves them beyond the complacent and routine. They have a clear focus but are not blind to the perspectives of others. They do not see themselves as experts, nor do they see parents as dependent upon them. Rather, they see themselves and parents as fellow human beings in a partnership wherein both they and the parents have something to offer in pursuit of the child's optimal health. EPPs deeply admire how parents know the child in ways that PHCPs never could, while they themselves know a great deal about the child's condition and the various forms of treatment for the condition. Recognizing that both they and the parents have the child's best interests at heart, they endeavor to work closely and respectfully with parents. By doing so, they acknowledge both the parents' agency and their own in making a difference in the situation. However, they also recognize that respect between EPPs and parents has to be a mutual relationship—from parent to provider as well as the other way around. EPPs' expansive way of seeing the world enables them to see widely and fully and yet, simultaneously, to focus, so they can select from a vast array of stimuli, elements, and details that are significant to each particular situation. They respect parents by purposefully looking at the parents' situation within the context of all that is going on around them.

Diversity as a Value

Parents did not talk explicitly about PHCPs' *worldview* or *values*, but they did allude to the positive ways in which EEPs treated families from differing backgrounds. For example, a non-English-speaking Chinese mother shared:

> Regardless of where we're from, we're treated all the same. It's easy to tell whether they've been fair since we've been in the hospital for some time. I've talked with some native [Canadian-born] families for whom I know the use of medication might differ, but the procedure of the treatment is basically the same. We're treated equally.

And an Indigenous mother discussed how one particular nurse's ability to connect with varying types of families made parents comfortable:

> She's really great at teaching and really great at communicating. She gets along very well with not just my family. I've seen her with other people and she's great with each different family. I don't know if adapting is the word because I know that our family and this other family are totally different types, but she gets along with both of us very well. She's great at doing that and then making us feel comfortable while we're with her.

What we did learn explicitly from interviews with and observations of PHCPs is that the scope of EPPs' worldview is global: They recognize diversity and view society as composed of individuals whose own well-being is inextricably bound up with the good of the whole. Their worldview of inclusiveness, interconnectedness, and perceiving that all human beings share a common humanity means EPPs welcome interaction with all parents regardless of how different parents may be from the EPP. Most often, difference refers to those who look or speak differently from oneself, but it also includes same-sex relationships, blended families, rural versus urban settings, or behaviors that may be viewed as outside the norm, for example, people who live alternate lifestyles or pursue alternative health-care practices. Such families present challenges for many PHCPs, but for EPPs who see these families not as problems or mysteries, it is an exciting opportunity to learn and to experience something new:

> There are a zillion cultures, there are lots of shirts. "Shirts" is a good word because you come from your background and I come from mine, but I think if nothing else, what I have learned—and I think that's why I'm still in this work—is that I appreciate all the different shirts and cultures. It's very interesting.
>
> I think it's neat, especially in this location where you get to see lots of different cultures. That's what's stimulating about the job, that it is so diverse, and I love the whole interaction process with different families, such as thinking about how you break bad news to different people from different cultures.

When the difference with a particular parent does present a challenge to providers, EPPs admit that they feel challenged, but they also do something about it. For example, when struggling to offer explanations to parents who have limited language or verbal comprehension skills, they may draw diagrams or use simpler words. They find a way to interact based on the parents' cultural backgrounds, but first they try to understand the family's agenda.

EPPs not only recognize difference in others but also acknowledge it. Betty remembers being in a cultural-training workshop where the leader pointed out that a person who proudly says, "I don't see color, I just see the person," is actually being dismissive of the other person because it is impossible not to see the color of another human being. Seeing and acknowledging difference while also recognizing the similarity between themselves and others means EPPs realize that the humanity of another cannot be divorced from their own humanity. Diversity then is seen as a strength, not as a source of avoidance, tension, or conflict.

EPPs are troubled when they witness inequality. They are distressed, for example, when they witness differences in the care because of who a parent of an ill child might be:

> We danced around and did all sorts of things that are not conventional with her child because she's a staff member and she had knowledge of how things worked in the unit. She was able to say, 'Okay, I want this, I want this. No, I don't want that.' But all parents should be able to say that and should have the teaching they require to say so.

EPPs demonstrate a sensitivity to stereotypical responses to, and interactions with, families who are different from them. They are aware of how parents who are different in some way sometimes receive less than optimal care:

> There are a lot of people having real hardships because of their economic situation or because of our presumptions about lifestyle. Do they get treated differently? Do they feel they get treated differently because they look different as one parent did, covered with tattoos and cornrows hair and muscle shirt? Yes! And they were the most amazing parents I've ever seen.

EPPs also feel distress with the relative lack of attention given to young, socially or economically disadvantaged, or racialized people. They note a lack of effort from some PHCPs to even go into the room, so these parents do not have as many opportunities to ask questions compared with the White families from wealthier backgrounds who are encouraged to not only ask questions but also make suggestions about treatments. For EPPs, such occurrences lead them to develop and practice the cultural advocacy, competency, and awareness skills with which they strongly identify.

EPPs note that clashes may occur when parents' values do not align with those of the medical culture and become evident when parents request accommodation for cultural practices, for example, an Indigenous woman wanting to have a feather with her in the delivery or operating room because she believes it is healing, comforting, and protecting, or Muslim couples expecting to have a female health-care provider deliver their baby. For EPPs, cultural awareness means understanding the cultural dimensions in a significant way. Such understanding derives from backgrounds that exposed them early to cultures beyond their own, which sensitized them to a range of cultural practices and enhanced their knowledge, for example:

> I was born and raised in the third world where there is poverty. You see poverty but you see love and goodness in the poverty. I also know the rich and I understand the poor, so I was able to bring those experiences together.

EPPs are also aware of historical aspects that help them in being culturally conscious. For example, an Indigenous elder who was visiting one of his families came into a social worker's office. His first words were that he had gone to a residential school[1] to which the social worker simply responded by saying *I hear you* and sat silently. She knew about residential school history and how it was the cause of survivors' deep lack of trust in institutions. After a full minute of the social worker respecting the silence and letting that information sink in, the elder broke the ice and invited her to go help the family. He understood that she understood.

Subtle signs of discrimination are clearly evident to EPPs. They are especially distressed when they encounter colleagues whose lack of self-awareness and knowledge about other groups is so profound that they do not recognize a need to overcome assumptions or stereotypes. EPPs' distress is heightened when stereotypes take the form of tokenism, which occurs when providers assume they understand patients' and families' unique cultural needs based on their exposure to members of the same cultural group, even though that previous exposure may have been limited or superficial: *I recognize it so much because I've worked on the reserves and in doing antiracism advocacy so many times, I hear things like, 'Well, I have three friends who are First Nations', that tokenism stuff.*

EPPs also seek to understand the larger, systemic implications of their work and have a critical perspective on their own cultures. In their work settings, EPPs care for particular families, but they also see the wider implications of their actions. They recognize how their work affects and is affected by the interdependent realities of their worldview. EPPs not only acknowledge inequalities, but they also take action to correct those inequalities, and so social justice is an important value for EPPs.

Social Justice as a Value

It can be difficult to spontaneously list your values when asked to do so, but in our study, values were clearly exposed—sometimes gently and sometimes harshly—in PHCPs' words and particularly in their actions. As it is for everyone, truths are embodied and values are represented in one's actions. EPPs' values keep them motivated, and values are key in what EPPs do because they hold everything together for the greater good. They turn to their values in moments of decision and for their actions that follow.

EPPs value social justice, which translates into a desire to provide equitable care for all, regardless of how different parents are from themselves. For some EPPs, seeking social justice is the reason they chose their profession: *There's never been a question in my mind that I would choose a career that would hold a place around social justice. I'm somebody who has an interest in supporting others who are disadvantaged whatever that looks like.* Other EPPs enjoy working in their particular location *because of our programs that seek to address the health needs of the population that don't necessarily have equitable access or equitable outcomes.* Earlier experiences motivate EPPs; for example, witnessing the disparity between the family of a well-off woman who had Parkinson's disease and other families without the same resources raised questions about how to address that gap. EPPs recognize social justice as removing the barriers that are the cause of such inequities.

EPPs identify the difference between equality and equity and recognize that principles of equity should be used to remove barriers and produce fairness. Equality is treating everyone the same and can be seen when PHCPs end up providing rubber stamp care that is outlined in manuals of how to interact with parents of particular cultures or in standards of care that aim to ensure patients receive quality and the same, or equal, care. But equality can only work if everyone starts from the same place and needs the same help, which is unlikely. In every interaction, EPPs practice from a place of cultural humility, and they continuously strive to improve their cultural competence. Consistent with the literature (Abdul-Raheem, 2018), they understand cultural humility as a process of self-reflection and self-critique that they need to undertake during multicultural encounters so they can accept and respect people of other cultural backgrounds, as well as the complexities of each individual. Similar to Cai's (2016) concept analysis of cultural competence, EPPs recognize that cultural humility is the foundation for cultural competence and that they can only develop their cultural competence through a dynamic process that includes cultural awareness, sensitivity, knowledge, and skill. Thus, they see and acknowledge that parents differ in many ways from one another and have different needs. Then, taking these differences into account, as well as recognizing existing structures of social inequities, EPPs aim to provide equitable care by providing parents with what they need based on their individual situation.

Family-Centered Care as a Value

Family-centered care is typically viewed as the gold standard of practice, and it is an expectation in pediatric settings. Yet significant barriers, including policies about visitation and clinicians' understanding of parental roles in hospital settings, may limit the full realization of family-centered care (Baird et al., 2015). Interconnectedness, however, is integral to EPPs' expansive worldview. They recognize that persons are part and parcel of larger wholes—their family and their culture—within which their life circumstances and relationships are intertwined. Everyone both is affected by and affects these larger wholes. As a result, for EPPs family-centered care implies that they must pay attention to the whole family as it defines itself:

> I look at the family as a whole, not just the child. It's the child and maybe grandma, or it might be mom and dad, but whoever is involved, I try to include them as much as I can. It's finding out from the family who's part of their family and what's important to them and their family.

EPPs are sensitive to how a family perspective is inherent in some cultures:

> The family is not just mom and dad and two kids. When we have large families that come here, culturally and ethnically they're connected and they're all wired together. For example, a mom is trying to make a decision about next steps when her child died and she's in shock because none of them were expecting this. The grandmother is the matriarch of this large extended family. There's no straight communication but there has to be a process of all this being worked through the whole family so the whole family is comfortable with it. Then, the mom can say what she'd like to have happen and it's something that she's comfortable with because she's talked with her aunts and her uncles and her mother. So, in such situations, I ask: 'Can we bring all the family together? Is everybody here that's important?' When I'm working with an Aboriginal family, 'Are the grandmothers here?' We need the grandmothers here because they're going to make the big decisions about certain things, such as about steps moving forward or even at times if there is conflict within families; when the grandmothers arrive, they settle it all: 'We'll do the memorial here and then the child will be buried over there.' Right, the decision is made.

EPPs acknowledge that family members affect one another and, thus, caring for the parents is central to caring for the child. They know that in family-centered care:

> You stop looking at the baby as your only patient—it's wider than that. It's making sure that you are not just looking at the baby's needs. You are looking at the family needs and by doing so, you are actually helping the baby too.

They also recognize that family-centered care is a two-way street because it is not just about serving the family; the family also is interacting with the health-care system. Sometimes, providing family-centered care requires creativity and advocacy within the system, for example, creating spaces with the proper ventilation so that smoke alarms will not go off when a First Nations family wants a smudging ceremony for healing purposes.

EPPs believe that parents' unique knowledge of their child is a valuable resource for optimizing all aspects of the child's care. They believe that parents are the people consistently caring for the child and are reliable observers of changes in the child. Moreover, it is the parents who have to live with the long-term implications of the decisions that are made for their child. EPPs believe that parents' input (thoughts, feelings, concerns, and ideas) should be actively and purposefully sought within the context of their relationship with the parents so that decision-making is a shared endeavor. EPPs are clear that family-centered care means parent participation, involvement, and decision-making, and that parents need to be part of the team caring for their child, not left in the dark.

At the same time, EPPs emphasize that a critical aspect of family-centered care is recognizing that their job and the parent's job are different but complementary: The providers have a broad range of clinical expertise based on caring for many children, whereas parents have in-depth knowledge of their own child. This differentiation between what providers and parents know means that the provider role has changed from doing everything from a position of authority and knowledge as an expert to instead informing parents and being a source of information.

Thus, EPPs believe that family-centered care is about understanding the parents' worldview and supporting them in their decisions and in their hope, even if the provider does not agree: *The family is usually right. I know that's a mouthful but if you think about it, the family is making decisions for their family. It's their child, not mine. It's their life, not mine.* Although EPPs believe it is their responsibility to foster collaboration with parents, they also note the importance of encouraging parents to be parents and not expecting them to be mini-nurses or mini-physicians:

> It's their baby and it's in their best interest to be involved, but they are still the family and we have to emphasize that they don't become little nurses and doctors, they are still mommy and daddy. They should not do our job; they should be part of our job.

Personal and Professional Integrity as a Value

Integrity is a value that allows EPPs to live their worldview. Moral integrity means that they know who they are and can be relied on to show moral character in everything they do. Being someone with integrity means that they are consistent in their convictions, actions, and emotions and are seen by others as being trustworthy. Integrity is important both personally and professionally.

EPPs perceive a shared humanity between themselves and those they care for, which means they need to have integrity. They emphasize the importance of having a high degree of integrity in their work and doing the best job they can, but they also recognize that they cannot always be perfect. EPPs advise to *always make sure you have your integrity. I never want to let my standards slip—that's important to me even though maybe I'm the only one who knows it. It gives me pride in my work.* Perhaps the key part of such statements is: *that's important to me even though maybe I'm the only one who knows it.* This very personal and reflexive component of how EPPs work is a major element of their practice. By looking inward, EPPs maintain their self-esteem. By maintaining their own integrity, EPPs' lives demonstrate a quality of energy and spirit that reflects the personal meaning they find in their work.

EPPs perceive their role as health-care provider as more than simply doing their job or carrying out specific tasks for which they have been trained. They aim to heal the whole person and contribute to the well-being of families and communities; they advocate for not only physical but also social well-being. EPPs see themselves not as experts with specialized knowledge and skills to fix others but as companions who walk with others on their journey. For EPPs, integrity is not the same as meeting another's demand for perfection in the sense of adhering to schedules or prescribed ways of doing things. Personal integrity has more to do with meeting their own standards for providing optimal quality care and finding satisfaction in doing so. Integrity occurs when the values in the care they deliver are congruent with their own values. A PHCP's behavior may fit with the norms on a particular unit, but that person may not have integrity. Maintaining integrity has to do with maintaining wholeness and being in alignment with their values about the right thing to do.

Personal integrity is being faithful to what EPPs say they will do:

> I always feel really, really strongly, and this is anywhere I've ever nursed, that if you say you're going to do something for families, you should do it. If I say, 'Oh, I'm going to be back in an hour,' or 'I'll be back in 15 minutes,' but if I can't get back on time, I'll say to them, 'I haven't forgotten about you, I am coming back.' Just letting them know you're there. This is such a huge rapport builder. This is in my personal life too: If you say you're going to do something, then you should do it.

An emphasis on being faithful to what they say they will do shows respect for others and helps to build rapport between EPPs and families. Owning up to an error and learning that they are not perfect and that they are not always able to answer every question but can find out all contribute to EPPs' integrity. Personal integrity is also linked to standards of maintaining commitments to patients that are often integral to professional ethics.

EPPs' worldview also incorporates their perspectives about and devotion to their own professions. They take their professional responsibilities seriously, but they also question rules, policies, and norms of practice. Professional integrity has to do with maintaining professional standards that are external to the individual PHCP, an idea that is captured in this way of explaining what maintaining professional standards is about: *I think there's your professional manner—your professional behavior and your professional appearance—and engaging in these things in ways that are not offensive or distracting in a negative way.*

Recognizing that parents of seriously ill children are in a very vulnerable position, EPPs aim to convey that they are there as professionals for the parents, the child, and the family. EPPs also realize that parents need to see how professional they are, so they create a professional appearance and pay attention to how they look. They know that *you can't look like you fell out of bed in your pajama bottoms, put on a clean T-shirt, and came to work.* EPPs are conscious of how exercising political correctness and general politeness play an important role in presenting as a professional in the eyes of parents. They also realize that professional standards may be different in other countries or even in other hospitals, so they are alert to what seems to be appropriate and what is not in their own setting. EPPs are aware that their own professional association puts forward guidelines for professional behavior that they readily access when questions arise. They also seek new information and insights by attending professional conferences or seminars pertaining to those guidelines. EPPs believe that a crucial part of professionalism is knowing what they are supposed to know and having the capabilities they are supposed to have.

For EPPs, maintaining professional integrity also involves interactions with their colleagues: *The professional part of it is just being really honest and frank but still respecting people you work with and not talking badly about them behind their backs, because this is a professional place.* When mentoring or evaluating students or junior staff, EPPs are honest about holding others to the standards that must be met.

As also identifiable in previous work from the early 1990s in adult palliative care (Davies & Oberle, 1990) and more recently in pediatric palliative care (Widger et al., 2009), personal and professional integrity are clearly important to EPPs. In our study, integrity was supported and enabled by EPPs' commitment to authentic engagement.

Commitment to Authentic Engagement

In most respects, EPPs are simply people who are committed to engaging as fellow human beings as the basis for their practice. We are talking not about commitment as an abstract term but rather as something that speaks boldly about one's intentions, that motivates actions that are stronger than words, and that enables people to practice what they preach. What a person is committed to matters, the content and the form of commitment matter. For EPPs, their commitment is to engage authentically with parents. This commitment is represented in our model by the hub of the windmill. The hub, located at the center of the windwheel, is the central point where all the moving parts come together; it is the connecting point for the wind-wheel and the rudder, for the gearbox and the central shaft—all of which are integral to the viability of the windmill. Similarly, for EPPs the hub represents the point where their worldview and values connect with an awareness of their direct contribution, both as professionals and as persons, to knowing parents as people and authentically engaging with them as partners in the child's care—all of which are integral to the viability of exemplary interaction.

EPPs recognize the interconnectivity and complexity of human relationships. As a result, EPPs focus not just on whether but on how they engage with parents. They strive to know parents not just as parents but as mothers, fathers, spouses, partners—as the people they are. Such knowing leads to a deeper understanding and appreciation of parents' life circumstances. EPPs can then offer help in the most meaningful ways: *My role as a health professional, as a healer, is to try to understand who you are and how you now respond to this thing that is happening to you.*

EPPs' commitment to authentic engagement with parents is manifest in authentic conversations with parents. The goal of their conversations is not manipulation of parents (to get them to make the decision a health-care provider prefers, or to change them in some way) but to get to the truth of the parents' experience, to share their own truth, and to talk together to reach a common goal. In our presentations about the model, some PHCPs expressed concern that getting to know parents in this way takes time away from an already always expanding, extensive to-do list. In contrast, because of their commitment to engaging with parents, EPPs choose to *make* time to spend with parents: *I think when parents are at their most needy and wanting information and wanting answers, to be there for them is really important because that's when you build relationship.* EPPs understand that every interaction, whether it takes a few seconds or several minutes, conveys a message to parents that either helps or hinders their sense of well-being: *It takes no more time to smile and greet a parent as one checks an IV than to scowl and say nothing.*

EPPs' actions are founded in their commitment, their passion, and their belief in doing what must be done, not simply what should be done. EPPs acknowledge that they are committed to engaging with each individual child, parent, and family, but that at the same time being committed to the individuals can sometimes be discouraging because it is so hard. Therefore, to carry through on their commitment, they have to be equally committed to the vision of being committed to others.

Although functioning in this way involves hard work, EPPs gently persist because they recognize a shared capacity for the feelings that lie at the core of an essential humanity: Suffering, fear, yearning, hope, joy, and love. EPPs' worldview and values enable them to see themselves as responsible for their own commitment and as the source of their motivation and morale. They work in committed and sustained ways amid the complexity of the institution, the health-care system, and society itself. They reflect the potential in all PHCPs to find the strength and quality of commitment needed to ensure that the human element of health care is not pushed aside by the advance of ever-increasing technology and bureaucracy.

Source of Worldview/Values and Commitment

No single event or life experience can ensure that a PHCP will or will not develop a broad worldview and its associated values or a commitment to authentic engagement. But several key factors can be identified as contributing to EPPs' expansive worldviews and ongoing commitment.

Experiences in Childhood/Adolescence

Childhood experiences helped lay a foundation for the global perspective held by EPPs:

> Growing up on the prairies really speaks to how I work, how I understand life. When you stand in the middle of a field of grain, especially barley or something with hairy tops, and the wind gets blowing and it's like a sea that connects the world—from growing up there, I very clearly understood that this is bread-making and the whole world makes a form of bread.

Many EPPs remembered growing up in hospitable places where their parents and/or other adults such as teachers, neighbors, or mentors fostered a sense of being at home in the world, a sense of it being possible to make a difference in the world as well as a sense of wanting to *try to meet people where they are at.* For some EPPs, it meant learning from observing the custom of hospitality that opened their homes and schools to the larger world.

Most EPPs' sense of compassion and justice corresponded to a parent's or their family's values. For example, the recognition of dying as part of living stemmed from an EPP's mother who:

> was really amazing about how she shared with me and my sisters about how to be with the dying. And I don't think that's very common, that people know how to talk to kids and know how to help kids about being with dying.

Other EPPs learned from helping their parents and grandparents care for a family member that the act of looking after someone who is vulnerable can strengthen and nurture the entire extended family, thus laying the foundation for valuing family-centered care.

For some EPPs, early experiences of grief and trauma fostered their worldview and values. For example, a traumatic memory about the medical care given to a young cousin who was diagnosed with cancer and eventually died led one EPP to realize that the doctors could have handled the situation better and made him interested in helping other families in similar situations.

Other EPPs learned from turbulent childhoods and lives of hard knocks that contributed to how they see the world and helped them develop a deep gratitude and ability to empathize with others. Yet other EPPs attributed their discovery of life's contradictions to being on the receiving end of injustice:

> I went through life in school with a brother who acted out, lots with the police. He ended up doing fine, but going into high school in our small town, I was identified with him with teachers saying, 'Sure hope you're not going to be like your brother.' I learned what it feels like to be labeled. So, at a young age, that got interpreted into justice work and advocacy and then in grade 12 to say, 'It's just not good enough that we keep doing this'.

These values are ingrained at an early stage in a child's life and may follow through into one's choice of career. Sometimes, these ideas consolidate very early, and a few EPPs seemed to have something akin to a sense of calling: *I've wanted to be a nurse as long as I can remember, like even 4 or 5 years old. I always wanted to take care of babies. It was my dream.* Though some older nurses made career choices at a time when there were really only three choices available to women (teaching, nursing, or secretarial work), even still they recalled deciding at a young age to be a nurse. Similarly, many physicians and social workers also remembered making their career choices early based on being aware of what they liked to do:

> 'I had a very high tolerance for children crying. I saw it as a challenge and I wondered how I could treat this child and get them to stop crying? I wanted to be a pediatrician from 10th grade.' 'I always had a little bit of compassion, a lot maybe, for people who were suffering.' 'I felt that my strengths were in compassion and heart.' 'I always liked the science behind it but also liking people and helping people and being able to make people better.'

Experiences With People Unlike Themselves

Being acquainted with people different from themselves contributed significantly to the expansive sensitivity of many EPPs. In their home communities, EPPs were familiar with their parents' friends or other community members who presented variability in age, occupation, social status, or cultural background: *I have been exposed to a lot of racism and poverty and things from my country's history. There are things that shouldn't have happened, but I gained a lot of compassion for people who are in a minority.* For others, living in or traveling to places beyond their own home introduced them to diverse opinions and lifestyles, such as one EPP who attributed their *love of working with people from different cultures* to having traveled a lot as a child. Another EPP remembered their experiences in Africa with international partners and how:

> people there did their programming while they were running from the Tutsis, meeting in a field in the dark to teach youth about agriculture. When I came back home, I quit complaining about my computer not booting up very fast. Not that I had to be African, but to really hear the privilege—even in all the advocacy—to hear the privilege. Those experiences gave me my holistic understanding of my holistic social vision.

Experiences With Role Models or Mentors

EPPs often remembered that exposure to a certain role or workplace situation as a student influenced their development of a broad worldview and values. A nurse recalled an early student rotation in pediatrics: *I saw how the nurses really got to support families, how much pride they took in helping families.* A chaplain commented that an early experience in a clinical pastoral education unit *caught my interest and I thought, 'That's something I can consider doing'.* In some cases, seeing a negative incident shaped and defined what an EPP wanted to do. A nurse remembered seeing a mother being taught improperly and being judged because of her marginalized status, which contributed to the child being close to apprehension by social services. This situation then led to the nurse's decision to work with this marginalized group of people and advocate for them.

An early positive experience was sometimes related to the EPPs having witnessed someone they admired in the particular role that the EPP was considering as a career choice. A physician remembered being inspired by two uncles who were physicians and how *exposure to these two people that I knew and trusted and respected had a big influence.* Some nurses too recounted being influenced by their mother or an aunt who was a nurse. EPPs remembered how role models or mentors provided examples of what it means to make a difference in the lives of others, to be open and welcoming to others, to talk about things that matter, and to learn what life is about. When mentors themselves have a broad worldview, are committed to authentic engagement with others, and recognize they are making a difference, they challenge, support, and inspire the younger mentee to follow in their footsteps. When EPPs are young and open to different paths in life, such mentoring may make a deep impression. But sometimes, EPPs also recognize the value of personal maturation as a prerequisite for understanding:

> I was really young; I was 22 years old. I think it's a lot better that I waited until I was older before I came to the NICU because I can't

even imagine myself as a 22-year-old having the interactions I have with parents now. It would have been so difficult.

With maturity and also the knowledge that came from experience, EPPs recognized and appreciated the abilities of some of their colleagues:

> I've seen some of what I call our exquisite providers where really, it's beautiful to see. I sit back and every time they engage with the family, the words they use, their physical stance, the way they use their eyes, their body—I just love watching how they relate to families.

When EPPs realize that they too, like their admired role models and mentors, are making a difference, they find work meaningful and they have a sense of purpose. They are motivated to carry on. This does not mean that they do not face obstacles or ambiguities; instead, they approach them as par for the course and keep on going, time after time, year after year. EPPs' worldview incorporates a long-term perspective that allows them to see themselves in relation to their work and their profession, and also to the society and the global community.

Ongoing Experiences

Finally, EPPs' worldview continues to expand, and their commitment to authentic engagement remains strong because once they find themselves in their field, they know that is where they belong. EPPs demonstrate an ongoing eagerness to learn more, for example, by identifying and attending conferences pertinent to their field early in their career and having their interest further sparked. EPPs express a desire to move forward and to do more; they need to challenge themselves. They simply enjoy many aspects of their work that others might see as stressful, such as being with children and parents during their most vulnerable times or enjoying defining characteristics of their particular setting: The intensity of the NICU, the long-term relationships in oncology, or the ability to help a child live while dying in hospice. EPPs are in awe of the strength, persistence, faith, and resilience of the babies, children, and parents. This awe is key to the ongoing enthusiasm for their work: *It was awesome to get to know people and understand where they came from. And I find it is one of the highest rewards to help a sick baby because you're really just giving someone a chance at life who has really not had a chance at all.*

EPPs also enjoy their social interaction with colleagues. EPPs are not lone wolves; rather, they have an interest in and a desire to interact with their fellow team members and to do all they can to make the team more effective. They respect their colleagues and, in turn, appreciate the respect they receive for the work they do: *I felt appreciated. Somebody recognized my talent and thinks I am good for my role and so I was even more committed and I worked harder.* Extending beyond their team, EPPs also perceive that if they help to make the system better, they are making things better for the parents and their children too, which in turn is gratifying and makes a big difference for them in carrying on in the larger picture. This sense of a growing satisfaction is vital to their conviction that they can make a positive difference—not just via their professional knowledge or skills, but via themselves and a commitment to engaging with others, human to human.

EPPs are sustained by the very processes that make them who they are. They have learned that they and the children, parents, and families they care for are all part of the fundamental interdependence of life. Knowing this truth, they cannot <u>not</u> act when faced with yet another set of parents who are caring for their seriously ill child. EPPs are devoted to being attentive to parents and faithful to engaging authentically with them. They convey not a sense of sacrifice or martyrdom but rather a sincere joy in how they relate to parents, children, and others. They sense growth in themselves and take pride in what they do. It does not mean that their way of relating always comes easily to them. They work hard at what they do, they encounter the inevitable hurdles that trigger fatigue and despair, and they recognize that this is a hard place to be and sometimes the people they work so hard to care for are:

> just plain difficult people. Or they're in a place that makes them grouchy, like a porcupine. But commitment needs to be married somehow to a principle of commitment from each caregiver that says, 'Well, even if you're a jerk, I'm going to take care of you.'

So rather than abandon their commitment, they find an alternate path to live it out. For example, one nurse described a practicum when she was in nursing school, working with ill babies, where she found she related well to the parents and felt a strong desire to work in a similar setting. Upon graduation, she was offered a job in emergency which she did not enjoy, and then by way of palliative care, she finally moved to NICU so that she could work with very sick babies and their parents. This nurse recognized that if she ignored her commitment to working with sick babies, her own integrity would be threatened. EPPs' work takes on intense importance to them, not because of any rules or guidelines, but because parents and children are suffering in the here and now and EPPs cannot look away.

Importance of Reflection in Achieving Your Career Vision

We are not naïve enough to think that everything we present in this book is all new and has never been heard before, though we do believe that we offer some innovative ideas. We recognize the work of the foreparents in every health-care discipline who had the vision to imagine what social work, nursing, medicine, and so on could be. But we also recognize that these visions, the ideals of practice, are not always the everyday reality in today's health care. We hope that our book can be used by PHCPs like you across the spectrum of your career, from initial education through lifelong practice and into retirement, to help you make choices that will facilitate meeting your vision for your career. So whoever you are, maybe a new student, an experienced educator, a novice, competent, or expert clinician, or an administrator, we want you to stop and consider who you want to be. To help you interact with others in the way our model suggests PHCPs should strive for, you first need to turn your attention inward—on yourself. You must first examine your own worldview, values, and the focus of your commitment.

You need to ask yourself multiple questions so you can identify who you are now, how you came to be who you are, and what choices you might make now, and in the future, to develop your career in a way that is meaningful to you. Start with questions such as: What is my worldview, and how did it develop? Reflect on your worldview and what you have learned through living your life by answering the questions in Box 3.1. Betty has had the privilege of working with a former research associate who has traveled to many parts of the world. In preparation for each trip, he learns the language of the country he will visit well enough so that he can converse with ordinary people on the street. As a result, he is often invited into people's homes and is immersed within the lifestyles of the local citizens. He returns home with a much-expanded worldview of how all people share similarities and differences and an eagerness to meet even more people and to learn more. Everyone does not have Betty's associate's linguistic abilities, but you certainly can aim to learn all you can from your own journeys to various sections of your own communities or country.

Finally, if you want to be a role model and mentor who inspires HCPs of the future, then you must examine yourself and what you portray through your ways of being in the world. Betty recounted a related memory that stands out vividly in her mind:

> I was co-teaching a second-year nursing course during which a colleague expounded upon the necessity of assessing the whole patient in preparation for surgery. She emphasized that gathering data about the patient's physical status was critical but so was assessing the patient's emotional and social status. To what degree was the patient anxious or frightened? Were there any social issues that might interfere with the patient's post-op recovery, such as had he recently lost his job so that financial worries might interfere with his recovery? After class, while our faculty group was meeting, a student tentatively knocked on the door and had a question for my colleague. The student's fiancé had broken off their engagement the night before and could she please have a 2-day extension for submitting a written assignment. Without

Box 3.1:   Worldview, Values, and Commitment: Questions for Consideration

Worldview

- What is my worldview, and how did it develop?
- What positive or negative childhood experiences do I carry with me, and how do they affect my worldview now?
- What memories from childhood and adolescence remain with me, and how do they influence me today?
- What is my perception of the world and the people in it?
- Do I see myself as an interrelated being with all other living things?
- How does that perception relate to my thoughts about providing family-centered care?
- How do I see my position of privilege in the world, and how does that affect my view of the world and all of its diverse peoples?

Values and Commitment

- Does social justice fit into my worldview? If so, in what ways?
- How was it that I ended up doing the work that I do?
- Do I have a passion for my work, for interacting with others?
- What is my level of commitment to authentic engagement with others? Have I even considered that concept before now?
- What types of people, or groups of people, did I associate with in my earlier life? And now?
- Who stands out as a role model or mentor in my life?
- From what do I find meaning in my work? Do I have a sense of purpose? What is it?
- How do I maintain my personal integrity? Is there tension between it and my professional integrity?
- Where have I lived? To where have I traveled? And, most importantly, what have I learned from those experiences?
- What have I learned about life and living from my contact with others whose lives are different from my own?
- Has my contact with others been only as an observer through the window of a tour bus? Or have I created opportunities for talking with people, for interacting with them in meaningful ways?

hesitation, my colleague curtly replied, 'You know the rules—you lose 10 points a day for each day of a late assignment,' and returned to our meeting. I thought, 'How do students learn to consider the whole patient when faculty do not treat them as whole persons?'

Who will you choose to be as a role model and mentor?

In this chapter, we have begun to point out some ways to use the model, but we would suggest that its use is only limited by your own imagination. We now turn in Chapter 4 to considering the process that underlies EPPs' interactions with parents and families.

Note

1. The government-established Canadian Residential Schools, starting in the late 1800s and extending for almost a century, were modeled on the Indian Boarding (or Industrial) Schools created in the United States. Similar to the United States, this network of residential/boarding schools was administered by Christian churches. The nominal objective was to educate Indigenous children, but the more damaging and actual objective was to indoctrinate them into Euro-Canadian and Christian ways of living so as to assimilate them into mainstream Canadian society. In both countries, residential schools have been associated with forcible separation of children from families, coerced abandonment of children's culture and identity, and sexual, manual, physical, and mental abuse. In 2008, the Canadian government extended an official apology to Canada's Indigenous peoples—First Nations, Inuit, and Métis—and instituted a truth and reconciliation process. The truth and reconciliation concept has been used extensively in Africa, Latin America, and other countries where restorative justice is sought to heal poor relations between groups of people—often based on the effects of global colonizations—such as White-Black persons in South Africa.

References

Abdul-Raheem, J. (2018). Cultural humility in nursing education. *Journal of Cultural Diversity, 25*(2), 66–73. www.tuckerpub.com

Baird, J., Davies, B., Hinds, P. S., Baggot, C., & Rehm, R. S. (2015). What impact do hospital and unit-based rules have upon patient and family-centered care in the pediatric intensive care unit? *Journal of Pediatric Nursing, 30*, 133–142. https://doi.org/10.1016/j.pedn.2014.10.001

Cai, D.-Y. (2016). A concept analysis of cultural competence. *International Journal of Nursing Science, 3*(3), 268–273. https://doi.org/10.1016/j.ijnss.2016.08.002

Davies, B., & Oberle, K. (1990). Dimensions of the supportive role of the nurse in palliative care. *Oncology Nursing Forum, 17*(1), 87–94.

Widger, K., Steele, R., Davies, B., & Oberle, K. (2009). Exploring the supportive care model as a framework for pediatric palliative care. *Journal of Hospice and Palliative Nursing, 11*(4), 209–216. https://doi.org/10.1097/NJH.0b013e3181aada87

4   Process of Attuning

Interacting is a bit of a dance—it's synchrony, attunement. It's like all those things that people talk about of what happens with a mother and infant—attunement, bonding. It's judiciously using your eyes, your body language, listening, being there, all of you in that moment.

In your everyday interactions with people—family members, friends, coworkers, patients/clients, and even those you walk by on the street—you are engaged in the complex social process of interaction: Navigating how, when, and to what extent you will engage others and if and how you will respond when they engage with you. Thinking of interactions as a social process may be a new idea—interactions happen so regularly, and often with such little forethought, that people often do not take the time to reflect on the steps of the process and how, when, and where they might intervene to modify the process and, in turn, generate different outcomes. Grounded theory, the research approach used in our study, offered a way to examine the process, as both a whole and in parts.

We learned that when EPPs interact with parents, they engage in an underlying core process that we have called *attuning to the particularities of the situation in the moment*. Six interrelated and recursive facets comprise this process: (1) *Orienting*, (2) *Seeking Parents' Perspectives*, (3) *Discerning*, (4) *Shaping*, (5) *Checking*, and (6) *Reflecting*. This process is represented in our windmill model by the blades of the windwheel. A key insight during analysis was our discovery that EPPs strive to engage in all six facets of attuning at the same time. It is not simply the case that the more facets you engage in, the better—nor can a PHCP excel at only one or more individual facet and still engage optimally. Rather, EPPs conscientiously, consistently, and simultaneously strive to engage in all facets while interacting with parents. Then the individual facets become part of the same whole: Just as the individual blades blur together when a windwheel is spinning in the wind, so too do the individual facets blend together into a cohesive whole.

Orienting

In health-care settings, orienting is most commonly used in the context of orienting new staff to the physical layout, the policies, and the procedures

DOI: 10.4324/9780429352393-4

of a particular unit or department within an institution. For our model, we use the word *orienting* to refer to how EPPs set the tone for their interactions with parents and for the type of relationship that follows. Interactions occur during different types of encounters, some of which address more serious topics than others. Whether encounters are planned or not, EPPs recognize that their body language, facial expression, tone of voice, and energy are all important because all of these ways of communicating your meaning are intuitively picked up by others. EPPs intentionally orient to parents in ways that reflect the EPPs' worldview, values, and commitment to authentic engagement, that is, *with their own selves and trying to be there as a human being.* For EPPs, orienting comprises three aspects: Preparing, setting the stage, and introducing oneself.

Preparing

Prior to meeting the parent face-to-face, particularly for the first time, EPPs prepare for the encounter. They emphasize the significance of not only gaining a rough idea of what the case is all about but also learning more about a family so that they better understand who they are going to meet— for example, where does the family come from? Are the parents married? Are there siblings? What are the parents' ages and occupations? In addition, EPPs use this learning as a means of establishing trust with parents: *I know who they are, why they're here, I've seen the X-rays. I give them a sense of we know what we are doing, that we know everything about their kid.* Knowing about the family ahead of time also enables EPPs to contemplate what they might say and do in the pending encounter:

> I also tend to draw on something I already know, particularly in a parent I've never met or if the child is complex—'I hear he's had a bit of a rough time,' and that always indicates that I'm not there just to do the job. That's part of orienting, letting the parents know that you have some idea of what's going on. Sometimes, I say, 'Gosh, it must be difficult for you—here I am, another new face—but I'm hoping you can catch me up on everything that's going on that I can't find from the notes.' And, if you don't do that, parents feel just like one of a number, and they're not.

EPPs may even check with their colleagues about what they think they will say during a pending interaction so that they can validate their plan.

When interactions occur spontaneously, such as during an encounter in the hallway or perhaps during an emergency, there is little or no time to prepare. In those situations, EPPs rely on their background and experience to guide their interaction in a *mindful* way. But even in such situations, the slightest piece of information, for example, *even if it's only 5 seconds with the nurse in the hallway who says, 'This is a family that has two toddlers, it's the oldest one that's ill, they're distraught'*, enables an EPP before they go in to mentally rehearse what they will say.

Believing that a parent's impression of a PHCP is largely framed within the first few seconds of any encounter, EPPs regard how they dress as a key component of preparing for an interaction. They emphasize that a professional appearance from the start facilitates the development of parents' trust. As well, EPPs think through how they will address each parent so that they can demonstrate respect immediately. In an initial encounter, EPPs address parents as "Mr.," "Mrs.," or "Ms. Surname" and then ask the parent about how they would prefer to be addressed.

Setting the Stage

Setting the stage for an interaction influences not only EPPs' ability to attune to parents but also the quality of the interaction. Therefore, EPPs seek a suitably private and quiet location so they can engage with parents. Further, they ensure that parents (preferably both parents and/or other caregivers as applicable) will be available and free from visitors or tending to their child so that a conversation can take place undisturbed and with the appropriate people in attendance.

EPPs also are aware that their own attitude profoundly affects the stage that they set: *If we bring an attitude of hurrying and busyness into interactions with parents, we show a lack of caring because it conveys, 'Don't ask me questions, don't ask for my help because I am too busy for your concerns'.* Thus, EPPs mentally check their own state of mind, for example, if they are fatigued, excited, sad, having a bad or a good day, or perhaps anxious in some way about encountering a particular parent. Particularly if they are not having a great day, EPPs think about that fact and they consciously work at being more mindful about who they are in that moment before going into the room and sitting down to speak with the parents. EPPs believe that when they are able to be in the moment with parents, then there are *more possibilities for things to happen that are good things around helping with symptoms, or hearing their story, or just being able to be more present—it's going to make a difference.* Consequently, to help set the stage for an interaction, EPPs take a moment to *ground* themselves by taking a few deep breaths, pausing for a moment with their hand on the doorknob to the child's room, or using other mindfulness strategies to help them concentrate on the situation. In fact, when EPPs make time to slow down, they become more effective. They find the time by simply pausing and giving their complete attention to the parent and to what is happening in the moment.

In today's world, people are accustomed to viewing time in measurable weeks, days, hours, minutes, seconds, and now, even in nanoseconds. Therefore, for many people time has become rigid and inflexible. This conception of time is reinforced when people's personal or work lives become a series of tasks on a to-do list. One EPP shared her strategy for whenever she is feeling rushed: She takes *a deep breath and says to herself: 'I have time'.* Her demeanor then becomes calm, her movements are unhurried, and parents and peers alike value her soothing presence. EPPs' attitudes and beliefs about time pressure profoundly affect their interactions; whether a PHCP made time or felt pressured by time influenced the quality of interactions. We heard about and observed many heart-warming, meaningful encounters between EPPs and ill children/parents that frequently occurred in brief moments, often because EPPs made time for them to happen.

Introducing Oneself

Some people may think of introducing themselves as a straightforward and relatively unimportant aspect of an exchange between PHCPs and parents. But we realized that it was not always done—we were repeatedly surprised at how often this simple act was forgotten or overlooked. Parents too frequently commented on how many PHCPs neglected to introduce themselves, and parents then perceived those PHCPs as *arrogantly assuming that we will know who they are*. In one case, family members had to assume that a particular provider was a physician because, despite checking on the patient several times over three days, he never introduced himself. So, without knowing who he was and because of his dour demeanor, they created their own name for him: *Dr. Grumpy*. Walking into a room without introducing yourself implies many things, but above all it shows a lack of basic social graces, which in turn implies a lack of respect that is felt by parents.

EPPs believe that how they introduce themselves to parents sets up a dynamic that immediately reduces parents' anxieties. Moreover, they maintain that introducing themselves is simply good manners or basic etiquette. They often shake hands and maintain eye contact as culturally appropriate. They sit to accommodate differences in height so that they can be at eye level with parents: *Sitting down when talking to parents is a doable, physical thing. So, the tall doctor hovering over a little mom who's cuddling her baby in the chair can maybe sit down to talk with her.* Such behaviors make parents feel welcomed, valued, and respected; these behaviors can be particularly important for parents whose first language is not English. When other PHCPs join a parent and EPP but do not introduce themselves, EPPs expediently and appropriately introduce the others to the parent or family. In addition, if other family members or visitors appear, then EPPs initiate introductions to ensure that the newcomers know who everyone is.

EPPs prefer to make initial introductions as quickly as possible upon a family's admission to the unit *before fears and challenges become an issue*. They purposefully introduce themselves to parents in a friendly, humble, and timely way. They do not rush; they take the lead from parents regarding what the parents are ready for. Recognizing that parents meet many people at the time of admission, EPPs try to be respectful of being *just another additional person*. EPPs consistently introduce themselves in very specific ways during every encounter with parents, and not just with a simple, "Hello. My name is. . . ."

How EPPs refer to themselves differs somewhat, but many use both their first and their last names, giving the parent the freedom to call them by whatever seems comfortable. They typically introduce themselves to parents with four pieces of information: (1) Their name, (2) their role, (3) their reason for being there, and (4) their availability. EPPs include these aspects in each encounter, recognizing that parents see a steady flow of people each day and cannot recall everyone. For example, on the first encounter, a nurse might say, "Good morning, Mrs. Jones. My name is Debra Eng and I am one of the registered nurses on this oncology unit. I will be looking after your son today and I will be caring for you and Kai until 3 p.m. this afternoon and then for the next two days." Having established a relationship with Mrs. Jones over a few days, Nurse Eng might begin to offer a more informal and familiar greeting: "Hello, Mrs. Jones. It's Debra again. I am back today but then I have some days off and won't see you until next week." Obviously, these introductions have many permutations and combinations that will vary depending on the particular EPP and the location of care, but the underlying purpose is to ensure that parents know who they are talking to.

EPPs mention their role partly to help parents learn about the various roles undertaken by the many PHCPs parents will meet and also to facilitate parents' comfort in an unfamiliar setting. EPPs believe that introductions should be caring in nature to help establish parental trust that their child will be safe and well-cared for. For EPPs, introducing oneself creates a human connection that is both personal and professional, implying competence and showing that they value social graces. Orienting, in our model, is the precursor to getting to know the parent, and thus lays the groundwork for subsequent interactions.

Seeking Parents' Perspectives

It is generally understood in pediatric clinical care that PHCPs must communicate clearly with parents to ensure that parents understand what is going on with their child. However, EPPs also believe the reverse to be true. They recognize that when parents feel understood by a PHCP, then parents are far more likely to understand the PHCP. Thus, EPPs aim to discover what is central to parents at a particular point in time, and they strive to get to know the parents so that they can fulfill their aim to engage authentically. EPPs seek information about a range of facts, thoughts, feelings, and experiences pertaining to the child, the child's condition, the family as a whole, parents' concerns and questions, and what the parents need or would like providers to do for them. EPPs' goal is to enable parents to tell their story. For example, EPPs want to be aware of the parent's understanding about what is happening to their child, to themselves, and to their family. They ask questions about where the family lives, what supports they have, if they have a belief or faith, and what they are most afraid of. They ask a lot of personal questions not to be nosy but so that they have a better understanding of the parent, because as one nurse said: *When I understand you, I can relate to you and I can give your child, and you, better care.*

EPPs also emphasize the importance of approaching parents (and others) with a recognition that any meeting is only a snapshot of a narrative, a value system, that has existed for years and is going to continue. Therefore, when they meet with a family, EPPs *want to get a sense of their narrative* because they realize that a family's story *influences all of their experience and our relationship.*

In seeking parents' perspectives, EPPs appreciate that their own expectations or perceptions influence the ideas they bring to the situation. EPPs are adamant that PHCPs must understand what families are going through and accept that families are often coming from a different place than the PHCP; so PHCPs need to put their own opinions aside. This approach does not imply that EPPs ignore or deny their own opinions or judgments. Rather, they are keenly aware of them and choose to put them aside so that they can concentrate on the parents: *Even though we all carry our own biases, we really must not judge parents and we must still assist them as much as we can.*

Seeing Parents as Partners

Underlying EPPs' approach to seeking parents' perspectives is their commitment to authentic engagement, their desire to develop relationships, and their appreciation of the depth and extent of parents' knowledge. They acknowledge that parents know every intricate detail of their child, and so parents are an excellent resource as collaborators working toward the health of the child. Because EPPs aim to create relationships with parents, they think of parents as partners in the child's care. At the same time, EPPs recognize that the power differential between parents and PHCPs is a potential barrier to developing relationships; so EPPs make a concerted effort to involve parents and to collaborate with them in decision-making:

> Ultimately, parents are the ones who know their child better than I ever will and so you need parents on board for the child's treatment, especially for stuff that is happening at home, like giving oral meds. So, you've got to make sure parents are part of the team. Because if you don't have buy-in from them and if they're not believing in what's going on, they're not going to give that treatment in the proper way. So, you involve them in decision-making upfront. Ultimately, they're the decision-maker for their child or the treatment. You have to keep them up to date. I tell them up front, 'I'm not going to hide things from you because you're the voice for your child and a crucial part of the team'.

Collaborating with parents as partners does not mean that EPPs simply do whatever the parents might want. It does mean, however, that EPPs take the parents' views seriously and discuss those views to seek a mutually satisfying conclusion. Yet, seeking parents' perspectives is sometimes challenging for EPPs. Some parents are reluctant to share their problems or ask for help (perhaps due to gender, cultural background, personal physical or mental health issues), or marital issues may be discussed by only one parent whereas the other does not see a problem. Other parents may present with *a sense of entitlement, that they should be given everything.* And yet, despite such challenges, EPPs gently persist, always staying attuned to the parents' perspectives, as affirmed by parents who appreciate that EPPs look at things from the parent's point of view. As well, EPPs develop strategies to help them engage with all parents. For example, letting families take the lead can be helpful; so they stand back and let families bring forward what they want to rather than try to fix things, because fixing is not possible. EPPs recognize:

> You don't know what else they have going on in their life. So you kind of try and talk about the care of their child, if something happened, and how to try and improve it or make it work for them. I think it's easier to try and just find out if there are other things going on. Being there for those parents to talk to and then sometimes it does help them a little bit.

Engaging in Two-Way Conversation

To achieve this partnership, EPPs *create a space* in which a two-way conversation with parents can occur. Many textbooks about communication offer guidelines for conducting focused interviews with parents or adult patients that will yield information about a pre-identified need that the health-care provider has in mind. Such information, of course, is critical to attending to the child's condition, but regardless of the focus of any particular interview, EPPs interact with parents by engaging in conversation wherein both they and parents can share their perspectives. If thought of as conversation, EPPs' interactions are then not about simply getting or giving information; rather, they are about sharing ideas, thoughts, and feelings to get at what matters most in this moment.

EPPs have multiple ideas about how to initiate conversations. One way that can be very helpful is to start with asking how much the parent or caregiver understands about the child's situation. EPPs suggested questions to prompt the sharing of perspectives: *After first explaining how you see the situation, ask parents how they are seeing it: How do you see your child right now? How do you see your child as different, for example, from this morning? From the last admission?* Also, EPPs open up dialogue by explicitly asking parents if what PHCPs are doing makes sense to them. And if PHCPs are fulfilling parents' needs or if there is anything else that they could be doing or that parents think they could do better.

Parents concur with this notion of conversation being of value: *Conversations with [EPPs] are much more of a give and take as far as spending the extra time to talk about what our needs and expectations are.* Additionally, EPPs' observations of parents' nonverbal behavior are also critical in enabling EPPs to *see if parents are anxious for their child, or if they are comfortable with where they are right now*. Importantly, parents' conversational and behavioral responses provide EPPs with clues about how to proceed, so seeking parents' perspectives helps them gauge where parents are at and gives them a platform from which to take off.

Discerning

Parents know their child's way of being in the world better than anyone, but having a child with a CCC means that they find themselves in need of specialized help for their child. It is common for these parents to feel threatened by things that other people do or say, particularly PHCPs whom parents often perceive as having much more skill and knowledge (and power) than the parent does. Parents' primary goal is to have their child optimally cared for. Yet, although they may not be able to articulate exactly what is at stake for them, they typically feel vulnerable when they first engage with the health-care system: *When first coming through the clinic, when parents hear 'cancer' they immediately think, 'Oh, my God! My child's going to die!'* Similarly, parents of infants newly admitted to the NICU are usually so overwhelmed that they do not even know what to ask. They are scared of the doctors, the nurses, and the environment itself. Though they may have some questions in mind, they cannot clearly express them because they are so scared and overwhelmed at first. Thus, in our model, *discerning* is how, through conversation and observation, EPPs try to understand precisely what matters most to parents at a particular point in time so that they can lay the foundation for a cooperative, collaborative endeavor to achieve optimal outcomes for the child and their parents/family. EPPs rely on interaction with the parents, and the family, to discern how parents are feeling and what help they might need. EPPs realize that often if parents need help, then their child also needs some help. So, they work together alongside parents and act on the parents' cues.

EPPs discern parents' state of mind or emotional status during each encounter because they realize that what matters most to parents at the moment is influenced by contextual and logistical issues that potentially interfere with a parent's ability to absorb information. Distractions from everyday life, such as financial concerns, child care issues, other family members, or personal considerations such as divorce or separation are all part of the situation:

> As you learn about all these types of things that are going on for this family—where they live, how many kids they've got, things that are important for these parents. They have five kids at home and now they've got this kid. Mom doesn't drive. How are we going to make this work? Because that's what will keep her awake all night. For me, it is important for her to know that we will make this work for her.

Discerning also involves identifying parents' strengths and using them to deal with problems, compensate for deficits, and overcome limitations.

Discerning parents' needs is an easier process with some parents than with others, even for EPPs:

> Some parents lash out at us or at silly things, like the color doesn't match the quilt. They'll find something small and lash out because they're grieving. So, you have to understand that you need to put your opinions aside and just listen to discover more about their expectations and reactions.

Such examples do not imply that EPPs ignore or deny their own opinions and assumptions. Rather, EPPs recognize their potential to influence the situation, and so they intentionally suspend their own views in order to concentrate on listening to the parents' story, even when it takes extra time. EPPs make the time to get acquainted and to establish trust by really listening to parents during their first encounter:

> I want to establish a solid relationship with the parents from the start. I do that by listening carefully to get to know where they are at. Some of my colleagues say that takes too much time but I would rather make that extra time at the start because then we are on the same wavelength and it saves me a lot of time later, which is important because I will be following this family for quite some time.

At the same time as EPPs listen and watch for clues about what matters to parents in the moment, they also are aware of their own values and what is important to them. They see benefit both for the parents and for themselves by getting on the *same wavelength*. EPPs recognize when the way things had always been done does not reflect their basic values and they then adapt to the situation at hand. For EPPs, discernment means that to recognize and sensitively interpret what matters most to parents in that particular moment they need to synthesize and sift through their own professional knowledge (e.g., about the child's condition and potential treatments), the information they obtained during preparation, the parents' perspectives and strengths, their observations of parents' behavior, and their own goals before they can then act accordingly.

Shaping

EPPs avoid reacting defensively or emotionally from a feeling of discomfort with what parents say or do. They do not stereotype or judge, nor do they offer some standard, pat reply. Rather, EPPs take the salient features of what matters most to parents in that moment and shape their response in a way that is tailored to the current situation. For example, although EPPs may enter an interaction with a tentative agenda for a particular activity, such as sharing the details of a treatment plan, they decide which aspects to discuss and which to leave for later based on their discernment of what the parent needs or can handle at that moment. They recognize that if parents are really distraught, then they probably should not try to give those parents a lot of information all at once.

Shaping is somewhat like improvisation—responding to a particular situation without specific or scripted preparation. In health care, ways of doing things generally evolve because they solve problems or make things more efficient and those things then become standard practice. Over time, many PHCPs become attached to those standard practices as the means to achieving what they were originally trying to achieve, but they also lose track of the original goals. Within their area of expertise, some PHCPs may be following best practice procedures and protocols and honoring the values that are obvious to them and their fellow specialists. But they may find it difficult to understand how certain practices are causing harm because their specialized perspective makes it hard to see what matters to others. This lack of insight exacerbates problems that arise in health-care environments that are complex and changing, as is the case when caring for children with CCCs. It is human nature to become attached to the way things are or the way a person does things. But once PHCPs realize that their standard approach creates or enhances vulnerability, they can also realize that it is better to put effort into discerning what they are really trying to accomplish and then shape their behavior accordingly.

EPPs appreciate the value of many standardized procedures or protocols, for example, related to activities such as diagnosing and treating the child's condition, maintaining a sterile environment to avoid infection, or controlling pain and other physical symptoms. But when it comes to relating to parents as the unique individuals they are and as one human being to another, EPPs are clear that standard or prescribed responses do not work. Instead, EPPs continually shape or tweak their responses according to what is most important to the parents in the moment. They appreciate the opportunity to figure something out and then, as appropriate, alter the words they use. EPPs identify what parents understand and reframe or rephrase things so that they better match the parent's understanding as much as possible. Shaping (and reshaping) occurs moment-by-moment and requires EPPs to see the whole picture while focusing on being present with one person:

> So somebody else comes into the room, the dynamic shifts and then, suddenly, what we're talking about may also need to shift. Maybe I need to sit closer or maybe I need to excuse myself. So you just constantly have to have those feelers out. I'm thinking of how the dynamics can shift very quickly. I am remembering one family in particular. When I first met this family, it was the mother and the grandmother. Later the father arrived and the dynamics were completely different. I think

it's about adjusting to the situation and if there's no flexibility, then you could be forcing something that isn't going to work.

EPPs need to have the ability to adapt based on what parents understand and need, as well as on the EPP's continual reflection during and after every discussion.

Shaping also has to do with EPPs sometimes having to intervene with colleagues, particularly for nurses with some physicians. For example:

> Some parents may not speak a word of English and some physicians come and babble and then leave. They seem to think that the mother's blank expression is "just" shock, or something—and then they just go. I have to interrupt to say, 'Excuse me, this family doesn't speak English.' Surgeons in particular have the habit of talking very "scientifically" and it sounds simple to them, but it's not very simple for parents. Most parents are not very scientific so providers have to adapt to the parents' language.

Checking

For EPPs, *checking* is not just about evaluating the success of a particular activity. Instead, checking with parents is being constantly attentive to what matters most to parents during and following an interaction. For example, evaluating the effectiveness of an intervention after administration of an analgesic to a child might mean learning that the pain has been lowered from 10 to 8 on a pain scale; checking is asking the parent (and the child) about how they feel now, given that the pain is at an 8. Checking also is a way by which EPPs follow through with their promises, for example, to find out more information or to drop by later. It was surprising and distressing to hear from parents how often PHCPs did not follow up on their promises.

Checking also contributes to EPPs' ability to prioritize the approach to use in the current situation as it evolves. For example:

> We hook up parents of palliative care patients at home with nursing support services. Some families want to go to the hospital, others want to go to the hospice, and then they change their minds and it's totally fine because the services are in place. We keep checking.

Reflecting

Reflecting is the vital sixth facet of the process of attuning. In reflecting, EPPs review their approach and a parent's response to what they said or did, consider their own personal reactions and responses, and identify how they might change their approach next time or stick with it. EPPs purposefully reflect by stepping back and thinking about what they are doing. EPPs ask questions such as: What happened here? What can I learn from this situation? Can it be done in a different way? Did I do something that I should try to better understand?

Self-Awareness and Responding to Triggers

Self-awareness is integral to reflecting because EPPs acknowledge internal signals (thoughts, feelings, or bodily sensations) that something is out of line and needs attention. Thoughts or feelings of not having done it right or well, or a sense of something amiss, trigger EPPs to reflect on those thoughts or feelings. Recognizing and acknowledging a trigger reaction, EPPs feel obligated to be honest with themselves and then take responsibility for their own behavior. For example, if EPPs have difficulty connecting with a particular parent, they would step back and ask themselves what was going on. They would acknowledge that something did not feel right and reflect on how it was their deliberate avoidance that did not feel right. They might then admit to themselves that they wanted to avoid this parent, so they would then know they need to work on understanding the reasons for that avoidance. When EPPs identify something they could do better, they seek to learn more; they want to change so as to optimally enhance their practice.

Reflecting also fosters self-awareness and discovery of how personal history affects EPP interactions. For example, one EPP had a father who always *told a joke as a way to lighten bad news for the other person, to make it seem less stressful than it was. I now occasionally explain to people that I too joke about things when I'm stressed.* For another, *it goes against my upbringing to ask questions, so I had to overcome this cultural pattern when talking with parents and learn how to engage with families through questioning.*

Sometimes in clinical practice, PHCPs realize when they have *reached their limit* and need to step back from a situation. But there is a difference between stepping back to avoid a situation and stepping back to reflect on a situation—the latter is what EPPs do. Avoidance is evident when PHCPs ignore their own triggers, or when they avoid focusing on the issue at hand. For example, in trying to rid themselves of grief and sadness, some PHCPs took a longer walk home and had a good cry to get it out of their system. But though this response is not inappropriate, it also falls into the problem-solving approach. It fixes the problem for the moment without reflecting more broadly on the PHCPs' beliefs about grief and sadness, their own personal history with grief and loss, how grief and sadness are dealt with within the setting, and so on. Little opportunity is created for new insights and learning about how to better handle similar situations in the future or to think about how to help colleagues in the setting who may also be sad and grieving. EPPs, on the other hand, recognize when they need to learn more, and they seek out resources, such as talking with a trusted colleague or with *someone outside of the work setting, like a trained counselor* who can listen to them and not judge them but really brainstorm about how to make things better and how to make it so that they can cope. Problem-solving deals with an incident; it fixes or corrects the problem at hand but it does not include thinking about what will happen next. EPPs go beyond the incident and are always thinking about additional implications.

We are not saying that other PHCPs never consider improvements. Indeed, other PHCPs may also sense that something they do could be improved; sometimes, they even recognize and identify it or have received feedback from others about a troublesome behavior. These PHCPs may even openly acknowledge the behavior as a personal limitation, but a main difference between them and EPPs is that these other PHCPs then allocate or expect someone else to make the improvements, rather than working to change themselves or whatever needs to be changed. As well, they do not take into account the impact of their behavior on others. For example, such PHCPs might admit, and also have been told, that their approach, especially when delivering bad news to families, is troublesome for parents and also for staff members. But they would simply state that they know they do not fulfill that role very well, so they rely on the team to do it. This "take me as I am" approach is not evident among EPPs. They understand that everyone has strengths and limitations, but they also believe that everyone should be willing and able to work on those things that are key to optimal interactions with parents.

Reflecting on Mistakes

For EPPs, reflecting is particularly important when a mistake has been made. They recognize that everyone makes mistakes and that when a mistake has been made, the PHCP should feel badly about it. If not, or if the PHCP keeps making the same mistake many times, then that person may be in the wrong line of work. EPPs strive to learn something from their mistakes so that they will not repeat it.

In contrast, in most situations when a mistake has occurred PHCPs typically tend to criticize or berate themselves for not following procedure and also attempt to fix the mistake by addressing the immediate problem. For example, imagine if a PHCP erred by giving a baby the wrong mother's milk, recognized the mistake, reported it promptly, and felt the weight of their mistake when the charge nurse advised that the physician and the parents had to be informed and it was the PHCP's responsibility to tell them. The PCHP might dread doing so but finds that the parents appreciated the honesty. The PHCP might be relieved because of doing the right thing—the mistake was reported and corrected. Problem solved? Yes, but the PHCP did not reflect on the situation in a way that resulted in a lesson for the future—the PHCP did not think about what was going on internally or in the environment that may have contributed to the mistake. For example, was the PHCP tired? In a hurry? Thinking about all the other babies that had to be fed? Was there something about the unit's organization of how babies were fed or about how the milk containers were labeled that contributed to the mistake? EPPs' reflection goes beyond focusing solely on the problem or behavior to be fixed; they uncover wider lessons that can be learned from an experience. In addition, reflecting by EPPs often extends to situations beyond themselves to identifying patterns in behavior among their colleagues. These abilities stem from EPPs' broad perspective into which their own behavior fits and within which they can see various patterns of behavior that have an effect upon the whole unit or on how the work is done within the setting where they work.

Reflecting can be contrasted with the normative pattern of PHCPs who when personally distressed by a particular interaction or situation simply recount the story of what happened without going deeper into the how and why of what happened. Standing at desks in patient care units, we (authors) have heard many a clinician's lament of exasperation following a particular interaction with a disgruntled patient or family member. The PHCP describes the event, releases emotions, sometimes receives empathy, and carries on. EPPs in a similar situation however, reflect on the troubling interaction and also on their practice in all types of situations and in relation to others, frequently asking themselves how what they did or what they said affected another person and what they could learn from it.

Reflecting and Learning

EPPs realize that the views they hold about others (their worldview and values, and their commitment) impact their everyday interactions with parents (and others) and, in fact, can either contribute to socially just actions or reinforce social injustices. Thus, EPPs reflect on the impact of their interactions in relation to their values. Such reflection also includes elements of curiosity and eagerness to learn more. EPPs perceive that reflecting contributes to self-care and personal learning:

> I reflect on and debrief my day during my drive home. Sometimes, I take care of myself by reminding me to be gentle with myself: 'You did the best you can, there was so much going on, you triaged, you dealt with the loss and that took three-quarters of the day, and that was good.' Reflecting has helped me learn to modulate my personality too depending on what's going on. In my natural setting, I tend to have an outgoing, boisterous, extroverted personality but this work has taught me another side of myself that I never knew existed. I'm much more calm, quiet, composed, nurturing because of the aspect of grief and loss that is here. But the extroversion works well if someone is trying to convince me of something that I don't believe is helpful for a family. So, I have learned to use facets of my personality as the situation requires—but it's all about advocacy for what's best for the family. As I have become more curious and knowledgeable and older, I realize I am continuously learning about myself—that's part of that reflecting process.

For EPPs, reflecting is made even more meaningful if done within the context of dialogue with others, for example, colleagues, teachers, mentors, or fellow students who are also interested in critical self-reflection about their interactions and themselves. They recognize that reflecting and learning are really important. When they work with students especially, they are constantly thinking of ways to help students learn from what the EPP has done and they often reflect with students. They find that sharing is really helpful because it makes them reflect on themselves and their practice, on what they are thinking and doing, and on what is working and not working with parents and others.

EPPs believe that reflecting is simply part of their job and they try every day to find some meaning in what they do. They often try to nudge others in the direction of reflecting, particularly those who seem not to have much insight into what they do. After interactions with others, EPPs think about the interaction and wonder how it went. They wonder how it was for the other person and if the interaction could have been better. EPPs have constant conversations in their head as they continually try to make things better.

Time for Reflecting

Finally, reflecting requires time, and EPPs devote not so much the time but the space for reflection to occur. Reflecting does not necessarily occur while EPPs are at work; it often happens later when they are removed from the hustle and bustle of the work setting. Because EPPs perceive reflecting as a necessity, they devote purposeful effort to the practice—it becomes a habit. They may not spend vast amounts of time at work reflecting on what they do, but they do take some time to reflect perhaps by going home and thinking about their day. EPPs find reflecting is helpful to them and has positive outcomes:

> Sometimes, in the quiet of the evening, things from the day come back to me and it's as though I hear a particular conversation again, with a wholeness. When I am in the conversation, I am focused on listening sentence by sentence, but as I think back over it, I suddenly perceive something—something that seems to be going on beneath the surface of the parent's comments that was never acknowledged. So, then, in that reflective space, I literally hear or see things as I'm thinking it over and I am open to the question, 'Was there something happening that I wasn't aware of?' This reflection is an essential component to my work with families and it sets apart this kind of work from a whole lot of other interviews where you are simply taking information and transcribing. This is much more creative and dynamic and I would say transformational.

The capacity to reflect, develop self-awareness, learn from experience, and fine-tune their practice and themselves is a hallmark of EPPs.

Further Thoughts on the Process of Attuning

Common to all facets of attuning is the ability to *make space*. Making space requires a simple pause, a moment to catch your breath so to speak, to center yourself, to ground yourself in order to really focus on the moment (Noble et al., 2019). A pause can occur in the midst of almost any activity—it is a suspension of activity, a time of stopping what you are doing, of taking your hands off the controls. It does not necessarily take a lot of time to pause—a moment or two, but maybe hours or sometimes longer as when you put an issue on the back burner for a while, or sleep on it.

EPPs momentarily pause before they enter a room to meet a parent; they pause when they are in the middle of a conversation with a parent, letting go of what they are about to say, in order to genuinely listen and be with the parent. They pause as they are weighing aspects that help them discern what matters most to parents and how to respond, they pause while following up and are surprised by the parent's distress, and, of course, they pause to reflect. Pausing means that the EPP is wholeheartedly present, attentive, and, often, physically still. A pause, by nature, is time limited. When EPPs resume activity, they do so with increased presence, clarity of mind, and sometimes, new insight. Of course, there are times when it is not appropriate for PHCPs to pause—for example, when a child in a wheelchair backs up too close to the top edge of the stairs or when a baby unexpectedly codes. EPPs pause to make space as a way of *keeping on top of things*. Doing so is largely responsible for their not being in a hurry even though they may have had a long to-do list and for keeping calm even when busyness flourishes all around them.

Often, you need to make a bit of space for yourself just when it feels impossible to do so—such as when you feel really angry, anxious when anticipating a potentially tense encounter, or overwhelmed by your seemingly never-ending to-do list. Although it may seem counterintuitive or downright frightening to do so, it is at such times that pausing serves a particularly useful purpose—it interrupts the flow of strong emotions and allows you to catch your breath and regain a sense of calm (Noble et al., 2019). Busyness is rampant in today's health-care system and in all aspects of life. It often stems from a personal sense of having too much to do in too short a time, which results in a free-floating anxiety that you are not doing enough to meet someone's (maybe your own) expectations, or that you are doing things wrong. Pausing creates space in the driven pace and habitual controlling of daily life where you can take a breath (and let it out!) and tell yourself that you have time. By doing so, you offer yourself gentle and non-judgmental support, which is the kind of support that EPPs offer to parents.

Exemplary interactions with parents require that you offer them this kind of support. To do so, you must engage in caring for yourself. The old adage of "physician, heal thyself" captures the notion that self-care, along with self-awareness, are among the components of exemplary interaction that all pediatric providers, not just physicians, might keep in mind.

Observing and Considering Attuning in Practice

So, how can PHCPs learn from others as they develop their skills in the *process of attuning*? What are some questions you might ponder as you think about the facets of attuning—related to both yourself and others? You might start with intentionally watching your colleagues as they go about their daily work as it is sometimes easier to see exemplary practice in others if you take the time to carefully observe and to reflect on your observations. Think about the ways in which you see others practice attuning and ask yourself the relevant questions in Box 4.1.

As well as observing others, you might think about the ways you can practice attuning yourself. For example, with *orienting*, you could consider your preparation and demeanor. One EPP was aware that his pleasant demeanor helped parents to see him as *approachable*, whereas another realized that her Spanish heritage of *hugging everyone and standing close to people during conversation* might not be appreciated by a shy, quiet-spoken, distressed parent. Like those EPPs, you might consider how to make efforts to reinforce whatever has a positive effect on interactions and to change anything that you recognize as having a more negative effect. For example, a social worker was aware that many parents assume that social workers are there because the family is perceived as having a problem or there is a concern about their parenting ability, so she

> tried to dispel the myth from the get-go by explaining that there were three social workers on the unit and they try to meet every family whose child comes to the unit because this is a very stressful time for them.

When *seeking parents' perspectives*, think about what you do to *ground* yourself before and during a conversation with parents. Some studies of physicians' interactions with patients and families indicate that the physicians speak disproportionately more than their patients (October et al., 2016) and are quick to interrupt patients' storytelling (Ospina et al., 2019). Do you think that you might also act in these ways? In relation to *discerning*, you might ask yourself questions such as how you figure out what matters most to parents. *Shaping* requires that you plan and adapt your next steps according to what matters most to parents in the moment, and that this adaptation is ongoing during all of your actions in this parent's situation. *Checking* or following up with parents is of great importance to parents. *Reflecting* is a

Box 4.1: Process of Attuning: Questions for Consideration

Observing Colleagues

- Who among my colleagues stands out for me as engaging in the process of attuning particularly well?
- Who do I identify as being an EPP? What specifically do those colleagues do that makes me consider them as EPPs?
- How and when do they *make space* before interacting with patients and families?
- Can I think of a time that I witnessed the process of attuning in action? What impact did it have on the interaction between family and provider? What impact did witnessing that interaction have on me?
- What, if anything, have I done to incorporate into my own practice the positive aspects of attuning that I have seen in others?

Orienting

- How do I typically prepare for a first interaction with a parent? For subsequent interactions with the same parent?
- How do I respond to the busyness of the environment around me and the parent?
- What does my body language, facial expression, tone of voice, and energy convey?
- How do I think my appearance may affect my interaction with parents?
- What does professional appearance mean to me?
- Are there specific things I typically say when I meet a parent for the first time? Do I need to change what I say?

Seeking Parents' Perspectives

- Am I aware of my opinions and judgments? How do I put aside my opinions and judgments?
- What approaches have I found helpful in encouraging parents to tell their story and share their perceptions?
- What is my view about working with parents as partners? How do I let parents know that I see them as partners?
- What are some ways I deal with the power differential between myself and parents?
- What do I find most challenging about seeking information from parents?

- In conversation, do I speak disproportionately more than parents? Interrupt their storytelling? When? What might I do differently?

Discerning

- What are some ways that I figure out what matters most to parents?
- What is it like for me when what matters most to parents in the moment does not fit with what I had in mind?
- How do I identify a parent's strengths to help deal with problems, compensate for deficits, or overcome limitations?
- Do I think that I am good at seeing the whole picture? What does the whole picture involve for me?

Shaping

- Do I consider myself a flexible person? What is my reaction to a change in the way I am used to doing something?
- How able am I to continually adapt or shape my responses to what a parent might want? How do I think parents see my degree of willingness to reshape my actions?
- How do I know that I have reached my limit? How do I respond? How does my response affect others?

Checking

- How do I balance checking with parents against feeling short of time? Do I in fact find that balance?
- What might I do instead if I want to emphasize checking within my practice?
- What promises have I made to parents and not kept? What happened? How did I feel afterward? Did I even remember that I had forgotten my promise?
- What can I do to ensure that I always follow up on my promises? Who can I enlist to help me when needed?

Reflecting

- When, where, and how do I reflect on my interactions with parents?
- Do I make the time to learn from my clinical practice? Or do I push thoughts of reflection aside and just continue with my life?

- If I want to incorporate reflection into my life, how might I do so?
- Remember a time when I made a mistake (because everyone makes mistakes!). What happened? How did I respond?
- Am I a different person at work than I am at home? If so, what do I suppose accounts for that difference?
- What are the stories that might have affected my desire to be a physician, a nurse, a social worker, a specific type of health-care provider? How do those stories resonate with how I engage with parents of children with CCCs?
- During my childhood, adolescence, or young adulthood, what experiences did I have in my home, school, or community that remain with me today? How did they affect my personality, my way of being in the world?
- How have ingrained messages or memories from childhood affected the way I engage with parents of children with a CCC?
- How would I describe my personality? How do I think my self-assessment compares with how parents see me?

critical facet of the process of attuning. Sometimes, people are aware of the deeply ingrained messages from their past that might be operative in their current lives, including their work. Other times, people are unaware of the influence those messages have on them, such as the impact of a character in a movie, book, favorite TV show, a memory (such as of a field of grain waving gently in the wind or a dying cousin in a hospital), or even expressions in the family that they grew up with, for example, a job worth doing is worth doing well, or the early bird gets the worm. If reflection is a new concept to you, imagine how you might be able to incorporate reflecting into your work. See Box 4.1 for appropriate questions to help you explore all of these facets of attuning.

Attuning is the underlying core social process of interaction between EPPs and parents. But our model of exemplary interaction encompasses multiple components. Reflection, along with the other facets of attuning, contributes to how EPPs approach their direct care activities—the component of attuning that is discussed in the next chapter.

References

Noble, H., Reid, J., Walsh, I., Ellison, S., & McVeugh, C. (2019). Evaluating mindfulness training for medical and PhD nursing students. *British Journal of Nursing*, *28*(12), 798–802. https://doi.org/10.12968/bjon.2019.28.12.798

October, T. W., Hinds, P. S., Wang, J., Dizon, Z. B., Cheng, Y. I., & Roter, D. L. (2016). Parent satisfaction with communication is associated with physician's patient-centered communication patterns during family conferences. *Pediatric Critical Care Medicine,* *17*(6), 490–497. https://doi.org/10.1097/PCC.0000000000000719

Ospina, N. S., Phillips, K. A., Rodriguez-Gutierrez, R., Castaneda-Guarderas, A., Gionfriddo, M. R., Branda, M. E., & Montori, V. M. (2019). Eliciting the patient's agenda—Secondary analysis of recorded clinical encounters. *Journal of General Internal Medicine, 34*(1), 36–40. https://doi.org/10.1007/s11606-018-4540-5

5   Direct Care Activities

It's our job to take good care of families, but caring is more than being technically competent. We also have to empower parents by teaching them, supporting them, guiding them, and being with them on their journey.

The blades of a windwheel spin around, but they have to be held together so that they rotate effectively. The stabilizing bands need to be strong to support and protect the windwheel's blades so that they do not bend, break, or fall apart. Both inner and outer stabilizing bands help to balance the blades. In this chapter, we discuss the inner band of our model, which represents the *direct care activities* that PHCPs carry out as part of their professional roles. It is during direct care activities that most PHCP–parent interactions occur. We will discuss the outer stabilizing band in the next chapter.

All PHCPs receive education in the various skills that are required for their discipline. Some of these skills are unique to a discipline, for example, the diagnostic responsibility of physicians, whereas others overlap across two or more disciplines, for example, how to regulate delivery of intravenous medications or how to engage with families. However, emphasis is sometimes put on <u>what</u> PHCPs <u>do</u> rather than on <u>how</u> PHCPs <u>are</u> in practice. Yet, as the EPPs noted, being good at the technical and procedural skills is not sufficient because caring also involves offering support to and empowering parents. The doing aspect is only part of what makes a PHCP an EPP.

Every encounter with parents triggers PHCPs to initiate direct care activities according to the obligations of their particular discipline. The predominant type of activity varies somewhat according to discipline, but in fact PHCPs of all disciplines engage to some degree in direct care activities during their encounters with children and parents. PHCPs talked about the various aspects of direct care that they give to children/parents, but only EPPs included certain types of direct care as part of their practice. Direct care comprises nine types of activities that fall into two overall categories of activity: *Doing-for* and *empowering*.

In *doing-for*, PHCPs use their technical knowledge and skills to do for children/parents what they cannot do for themselves. In *empowering*, PHCPs

DOI: 10.4324/9780429352393-5

help parents do for themselves what they want or need to do for their child or for themselves. Interactions with parents are inherent in both realms of direct care activity, but interaction is integral to empowering whereas, as parents and some PHCPs reported, doing-for activities can be carried out with little attention to interaction.

Transitions

The extent to which families require emphasis on doing-for or empowering activities depends upon where they are in the many transitions that occur over the course of the child's condition, for example, the transition at the time of diagnosis or when there is a change in treatment pattern. We found that parents and PHCPs alike described a similar pattern of parental response to every change, even seemingly minor ones, in their child or in the situation: Parents were initially shocked and distressed, then they were in a place filled with sadness, despair, and uncertainty, and then, finally, they were able to take a deep breath and move on to what needed to be done. This pattern of response is akin to Bridges and Bridges' (2019) concept of transition that has relevance to individual transitions. Bill Bridges proposed that transitions trigger a three-step process that begins with an ending (when a change has occurred), enters a mid-phase that he called the "neutral zone," and ends with new beginnings, which brings to mind T. S. Eliot's famous words: "What we call the end is often the beginning/and to make an end is to make a beginning/the end is where we start from."

For parents, the start of a transition occurred when a place of certainty ended, seemingly quickly, and triggered an ending of something that had seemed stable or secure. For example, bad news about a diagnosis of serious illness, their child's relocation to another facility, or postponement of a long-awaited appointment suddenly turned their lives upside down. Thoughts flooded their minds: What will we do now? How are we going to manage? What does this mean? Questions and ideas abounded along with strong emotions of shock, anger, frustration, and distress.

Parents then entered a middle, or neutral, zone where they felt they no longer fit with the past because the certainty they thought they had, the familiarity they had felt, was gone. They also felt disconnected from the present and the future seemed impossible. Bridges and Bridges (2019) described this middle zone as similar to being in a car that is in neutral gear—no matter how heavily you press the gas pedal, the car moves neither forward nor backward. This middle zone is a place of inaction, despair, distress, and worry—it can be a frightening and disconcerting place; you are simply stuck with myriad thoughts and feelings that weigh heavily. In contrast to the suddenness of the first phase, this middle phase seems slow and heavy.

But being slow for a time allowed parents to get their bearings once again. Thoughts, ideas, concerns, and realities settled down—parents were able to take a deep breath, realize some clarity about what now needed to be done in light of the changed situation, and begin again. They were ready to learn new skills, make a decision, and plan. Parents then forged on until the next transition was thrust upon them, for example, by another bit of disconcerting information. Regardless of parent or trajectory variations, PHCPs sought to achieve the best possible outcome for all parents.

Doing-For Activities

Doing-for activities are: (1) *Administering Treatments or Carrying Out Procedures*, (2) *Attending to Physical Care*, (3) *Managing Technology*, (4) *Seeking Consultation From Other Professionals*, and (5) *Referring to Other Services*. These behaviors encompass the technical or hands-on clinical skills that PHCPs, particularly nurses, physicians, and various therapists (e.g., respiratory) are taught from the start of their educational programs. There is no doubt that these skill-based activities are crucial and mandatory for PHCPs because technical proficiency is required for clinical competence. However, we focused on interactions in our study and not on assessing the competency of PHCPs, and so we are not discussing specific doing-for activities in this book. However, parents frequently commented on how well PHCPs carried out doing-for activities. In fact, parents' observations about a PHCP's technical expertise in caring for not only their own infant or child but also for other children/parents was how parents determined whether PHCPs knew what they were doing. It is no wonder then that expertise and speed in *administering medications or treatments, attending to physical care*, or *managing technology* may have become a source of PHCPs' professional identity and self-esteem. Indeed, the tendency was for direct care activities to comprise PHCPs' daily to-do list, a series of tasks to be completed quickly and well. Focusing on this list of tasks was expressed in an attitude of busyness and hurry and, even though the activities may have been carried out with remarkable technical skill, they also may have been done with what parents perceived as *impersonal detachment*, an approach that parents were sometimes willing to tolerate for the sake of PHCP technical competence.

For parents, competency meant that PHCPs were doing things properly, carefully, gently, and effectively. They were also efficient—that is, competent PHCPs were able to get done what needed to be done for a particular task or within the time allotted to them; they avoided mistakes. They were comprehensive, thorough, and *like good flight attendants, they cross-checked the doors*. Competent PHCPs were also straightforward and direct when they communicated about what they were doing and why; they got to the point. They knew what they were doing; they were *no nonsense*. Witnessing PHCPs who were competent gave parents a sense of safety, comfort, and reassurance; they were not worried because their child was in skillful hands and they felt that their child would be well cared for.

EPPs realize and respect that parents do not automatically trust PHCPs and, similar to parents, they believe that giving safe care is a requirement for competence, which in turn is a requisite for trust: *Pediatric health care providers have to prove themselves worthy of parents' trust and create a trusted environment for families where high-quality safe care is provided for the child.* EPPs also describe competence as *not making a mistake, such as a medication error,* and so they need to be able to focus, concentrate, and not be distracted: *If I am changing intravenous lines, I don't want to have a conversation with anyone unless it's absolutely necessary.* EPPs ensure safety by recognizing their limitations and not hesitating to ask for whatever they need to be sure they are doing things right and giving safe care: *I don't care if I look stupid by asking questions. If I don't know something, I will find the best practitioners to give me the answer to the problem that I have.* EPPs also demonstrate competence by *being as organized as possible in a chaotic environment.*

Some parents equated competency with experience, differentiating between seasoned professionals and *rookies.* When parents asked questions or when things happened, they described rookies as *like a deer in headlights,* neither knowing nor noticing. Rookies had little experience in the unit or in doing something on their own. Parents expressed concern that if one rookie followed another one on a subsequent shift, care and parents' confidence deteriorated.

Parents were adamant that PHCP skills must be matched with the complexity of care needed by the infant or child. Similarly, PHCPs believed that provider skills should match the situation. So, for example, when float nurses came to oncology, the implication was that those nurses may not be as well-prepared as oncology nurses and so their level of care might be less than that of oncology nurses or that there were things happening that those float nurses would not understand. Administrators also recognized these challenges and tried their best to match PHCPs' skill set with patient needs.

EPPs articulate additional components of competence, such as noting how competence is related to *a solid knowledge base as well as professionalism.* Further, competence is *not being offensive in dress or manners, as well as knowing what you are supposed to know and having the capabilities you're supposed to have in that role.* EPPs indicate that competence is not just *using the right skill at the right time with the right patient, because what matters is the provider who is using the skills.* Thus, EPPs include interactional skills in their connotation of competence. Therefore, EPPs not only engage competently in doing-for activities but they also give equal, or sometimes even greater attention to, their personal interactions with parents—these clinicians are the providers parents describe as excellent or exemplary.

Seeking consultation from other professionals and *referring to other services* both involve PHCPs interacting with other professionals on behalf of the ill child and parents. In doing so, EPPs again pay close attention to not only the technical or clinical facts of the situation but also the nature of their interactions with colleagues. EPPs recognize that though being highly competent in technical skills is necessary for PHCP excellence, technical competence alone is not sufficient for a particular PHCP to be described as exemplary.

Rather, EPPs understand that both technical and interactional skills are necessary for competence. Empowering direct care activities are entirely dependent upon PHCP interactional abilities.

Empowering Activities

Empowerment is a process that takes time, so it is not a one-time or a quickly achievable goal. Empowering activities are: (1) *Navigating*, (2) *Supporting*, (3) *Sharing Information*, and (4) *Teaching*. EPPs use the word *empower* to describe interactions with parents that aim to enhance parents' capacity to face and deal with the challenges of a seemingly overwhelming situation. To achieve this goal, EPPs facilitate parents' comfort in the setting and help parents learn to do all that they can for their child. EPPs deem that empowering parents also has the practical effect of optimizing care and perhaps even expediting discharge. For EPPs, empowering parents is a high priority: *The best thing you can do for a family is to empower them.* Such a comment derives from EPPs' broad perspective on the human condition and on human capacity, believing that there is almost nothing parents cannot learn to do. EPPs believe that parents know their child best, that they need to be well-prepared for managing their child's care when (and if) the child goes home, and that parents are, in fact, the ones who have the right to care for and make decisions about their child's care. Consequently, EPPs trust that parents are more than capable of caring for their children.

However, not all PHCPs share such thoughts because they do not trust parents enough to *allow, not even to encourage* them to be involved in their child's care. Some PHCPs resist allowing a parent to do something that only a *professional should be doing*, such as taking an infant's temperature, because the *baby is too sick* or the *parents are afraid.* Yet, EPPs believe that parents should be encouraged to be *hands-on as soon as they can* because if parents are more involved earlier, then they are ready to take their child home sooner. EPPs also indicate that parents of premature or really sick babies need additional emotional support and communication. So rather than PHCPs being *busy with the baby,* they need to interact more with the parents and carefully answer a parent's question because those parents require a lot of explanation about what is going on. Of note, such comments came from NICU nurses, so their observations may apply to NICU in particular, especially because a nurse in oncology referred to how parents in that unit were well-prepared to care for their ill children: *Parents from oncology know how to give medications, take care of IVs and central lines. They know how to do tube feedings, how to do pretty much everything. We empower them to take care of things right away.*

Empowerment as a concept makes some PHCPs uncomfortable: *Parents end up being the leaders almost and they end up dictating the care*, parents *overstep their boundaries.* This choice of words and language indicates clear parameters in terms of what parents should and should not do, what they are able to dictate, and what is off limits. This approach is quite the opposite of empowerment. Placing restrictions and perhaps even resenting those parents who do things that *compromise our care* indicates a non-collaborative, perhaps even a confrontational, stance. Such PHCPs may be unsure of the whole process of empowerment and find it difficult to articulate what empowerment means. That perspective stands in contrast to the way EPPs describe empowerment—as a process that is achievable, doable, and valuable. In fact, EPPs equate empowerment with the parents being part of the team; so EPPs strive to involve parents as soon as possible and ensure they are present when decisions are being made. The process of shared decision-making can be complicated, especially where there are competing interests, for example, when parents are divorcing or insisting on alternative opinions, but EPPs can help work through these challenges and help everyone achieve consensus. So even under trying circumstances, parents can be empowered and involved in the process of planning care. Specific empowering activities are *navigating, supporting, sharing information,* and *teaching.*

Navigating

EPPs' broad perspective of the world enables them to appreciate the complexity and interrelatedness of many aspects of a situation. Thus, EPPs appreciate how all aspects of parents' lives are turned upside down when their child has been diagnosed with a CCC and admitted for care. EPPs understand that parents need time as they ponder their changing circumstances and every new bit of information, struggle with a multitude of questions and concerns, grapple with mystery, and feel lost, anxious, and confused. Families need help to adjust to the diagnosis, to what it means to have a child with a CCC. EPPs see their role as helping parents as gently as possible to see the big picture, to deal with the multiple issues that come up that often leave families feeling out of control.

Moreover, it is not just at the critical time of admission but also throughout a child's trajectory, such as whenever a new crisis occurs, that EPPs feel responsible for guiding or *navigating* parents to help them through this *foreign land with its own culture and language and where seemingly simple things often assume complicated dimensions.* EPPs purposefully navigate parents through the setting, its procedures, routines, and people. Starting with how PHCPs orient themselves during introductions, as discussed in Chapter 4, parents appreciate being told who is who and who does what on the unit because this knowledge helps them know *who to ask, what to ask, when to ask it, and how to ask a question.* Parents are comforted by just knowing things like how to find their way to the cafeteria.

Most parents did not know what they did not know, so they could not ask questions or they were timid about bringing up relatively *unimportant* concerns. If they arrived from out of town, they were often even less aware of some basic day-to-day aspects of life in the city, such as how to use the city bus system. Both EPPs and parents frequently noted that parents did not know certain services were available and only slowly learned on their own about logistical issues and about the resources available to them, for example, how and where to park, how to efficiently get from one place to another, and how to access financial-aid programs. Because navigation was left to each PHCP to do in an informal way, some parents learned to navigate the system, or only some aspects of it, and other parents did not. Thus, many parents turned to other parents for guidance, but one parent's experience is not always accurate or applicable to another parent's situation. So some EPPs have their own way of navigating families around how to deal with the amount and type of information they receive from other parents, for example:

> I say to them it's a little bit like having a baby—everybody has a horror story to tell you how bad it is. Parents are well-meaning, but if they scare you or they say something, you have to come and ask me about it because they're all different—different treatment, different diagnoses, and different diseases. But these families all become part of a new club and they want to sort of initiate the new ones into what cancer means for them.

Navigating, therefore, also involves correcting parents' misconceptions that contribute to their challenges and fears. For example, a parent whose daughter was being considered for transfer to the hospice for respite exclaimed, *We're not ready to leave her!* This parent's impression was that parents could not stay with their child in the hospice but the hospice nurse explained otherwise: *You don't need to leave her. If there's a family suite available, you can actually stay in-house and for the first few admissions you could stay until you get to know the place.* Misconceptions mean that often families are really afraid to go to hospice, especially if they believe that the hospice means only end-of-life care and the child is going to die.

Though EPPs did their best to guide parents, navigating overall seemed somewhat haphazard in how it was carried out, and it also varied by location. For example, on admission to the NICU, parents initially found it to be a chaotic environment where they had to quickly learn many new things and meet many people. Some parents were *in chaos at first* and only learned about the setting *via trial and error and happenstance,* all of which consumed a lot of energy that would have been better spent in dealing with the pervasive fatigue that these parents often felt. Social workers were particularly good at navigating for parents, but during the conduct of our study the NICU had only two part-time social workers who connected with families more on an as-needed basis due to the large population on the unit. In oncology, on the other hand, each family was assigned a social worker as part of the primary care team for the family.

Parents strongly advised that they should receive navigation as soon as possible following admission. They suggested that one person should be specifically assigned as the navigator for all parents, rather than it being left to each PHCP. They also suggested that information about day-to-day activities and policies, such as visiting policies, be provided in both written form (brochures, handouts) and online, as well as in a variety of languages. Parents emphasized that this material should be intentionally given to parents on admission—not just left available on a table for discovery by happenstance. Such information needs to go to all parents and even more so for parents whose first language is not English or who are unfamiliar with hospital culture. EPPs agree and also note that such information would be helpful for new staff and students too.

Supporting

EPPs believe that *supporting* families is an integral component of their professional role: *I think that physicians and nurses in general, and social workers in particular, know that their role is to support. When I'm taking care of a family, I'm there to help them. So that's what my job is.* They value the cerebral aspect of interactions with parents, for example, discussing the diagnosis and treatment, but they also value providing support.

Supporting behaviors are particularly evident in EPP interactions with parents who are in the in-between space of knowing and not knowing, of having information but not yet knowing what it really means or what to do about it, that is, in the neutral zone of transition. Parents in this in-between place are asking questions and with support *they accept that maybe there isn't an answer today but we're having a conversation and there might be an answer tomorrow.* EPPs describe supporting as walking alongside parents until they are able to keep going by themselves or until something changes inside them that makes them more accepting of the situation. EPPs support parents by making sure they answer questions and by trying to make an awful situation a little more bearable, a little less overwhelming, for example, when parents are waiting for tests results, which is often really scary, or when they are upset.

While in the neutral zone, parents are on an inner journey that they alone have to travel. But they appreciate being accompanied by someone to whom they can express what they are thinking and feeling, someone who does not judge or evaluate them but accepts whatever is happening in that moment. Parents value talking to somebody who is not family and getting an outside perspective on whatever is worrying them. Sometimes parents just need to cry or be angry and *have someone hear them or they're just going to blow because they can't hold it all in.* Supporting sometimes means advocating for parents without judging, for example, honoring a parent's wishes by telling the team that the parent does not want anyone to mention hospice:

> I felt like I could be an advocate for that parent. It was a good example of honoring a parent where they're at. It's hard because there's so much

judgment about where these families are at. But we don't have the right to jump in and say they're not coping, or they are.

Advocating for parents in this way requires that EPPs suspend their own opinions and empathize with the parent. Support through advocacy also means speaking up for parents who do not have a voice:

> I find often it's the families who are the least demanding who don't always have a strong voice and I have a very strong voice. I chose a family yesterday that is just the opposite of me. The mom is incredibly shy, not particularly well-educated, and English is not her first language. But I know someone must speak for her and that medical staff, my fellow colleagues, won't overlook me. If I want something for 'my' family, I'll get it.

EPPs support families by staying with them when they are at their most vulnerable, such as when a child is approaching death. Parents were sometimes surprised by how an EPP stayed with them at that time. Upon hearing the nurse say they were glad to be on shift during the time the child was dying, a parent said: *Oh, she's so near the end—I thought you wouldn't want to have her.* But supporting is also *being with parents as they grapple with the mystery of life and death* because parents <u>now</u> *want to know how to think about death. Maybe they've never had a reason to really go there or think about how they understand themselves in this moment, in this world with all the mystery.*

EPPs also recognize that it is within the neutral zone where parents weigh pros and cons, struggle with what to do, and eventually come to a decision. However, EPPs do not regard decision-making as a procedure, as a cognitive process of measuring out the pros and cons that clearly point the way, as something that can be done using a problem-solving approach, or as something that with concerted effort can be done efficiently and quickly. Rather, an EPP's approach illustrates the maxim that life's most important decisions are discovered, not made. The neutral zone is a place of uncertainty, not yet a place of clear direction. Only with time, talking things over with someone who really listens, and receiving some encouragement or possibilities to mull over do parents begin to think about what will happen next as they find themselves ready to start a new beginning:

> Okay, if my child needs this particular treatment, then what do we do about it? If I am supposed to learn how to care for this trach, then how do I do that? If my child can no longer stay in the hospital, where else can we go and how do we get there?

EPPs recognize that parents are the decision-makers for their children and that the EPPs' job is to support parents during this process whether they agree with the decision or not. EPPs take pride in how well they engage with families when there is a decision to be made and in their support of parents regardless if parents choose to withdraw care or not.

From the outside looking in, the activity of supporting parents can appear to others as if nothing is happening. However, supporting parents involves considerable work as EPPs are always thinking, asking questions, or probing gently about what is central to the parent in the moment. EPPs are actively engaged even if they do not seem to be doing anything in the sense of being busy. The nature of the neutral zone is that parents are slowed down, even if sometimes only for a short time, but their sense of time shifts as they ponder so much new information, struggle with a multitude of questions and concerns, feel lost and confused, and grapple with mystery. PHCPs who are in *the fast lane, or who cannot or have trouble slowing down* often have difficulty offering support. In contrast, EPPs who *slow down to just be with parents, to offer comfort* empower parents to do what has to be done.

Sharing Information

For EPPs, central to empowering parents is ensuring that they are well-informed. Providers and parents indicated that the focus of most PHCP–parent interactions is the giving and receiving of information about the child's condition, treatment, and care, including diagnosis, prognosis, and end-of-life issues, about the factors that influence these areas, about the child's daily life in the setting, about the parents' life in the setting, and about procedures that the parents have to learn to do. Indeed, parents had much to say about information.

Parents indicated that not only <u>what</u> information they receive is important but so too is <u>how</u> information is given to them. What parents desired was accurate information about what was happening and what to expect. They wanted to know what the next few steps would be, what they would be doing next. Parents wanted signs and symptoms explained or interpreted so that they could understand, for example, *There has been a brain bleed but we now know that with physio and rehabilitation, the consequences are not as serious as they once were.* In particular, most parents were annoyed with hearing about percentages and acronyms unless they were explained, for example, that *there's a 60% chance the PDA (patent ductus arteriosis) will close.* They wanted to know what it meant specifically for their child.

With regard to how information was given, parents appreciated the use of simple language rather than jargon or anatomical, clinical, or surgical descriptions that were beyond their comprehension. They valued PHCPs whose approach was gentle, kind, sensitive, and polite, who *look at the parents rather than at their own hands or notebook*, and who take into account what parents know and think. PHCPs who parents rate highly in this regard are perceived as EPPs because they facilitate two-way conversations in which they and the parents are mutually engaged; the interaction is not solely about giving information but rather it is about sharing an experience of exchanging information. Underlying this approach is EPPs' viewing themselves not just as experts delivering information to parents, but as companions on a shared journey with parents wherein both they and the parents have information to share and discuss.

To facilitate this kind of interaction, EPPs create a context or a space for asking and answering questions that enhances understanding by both themselves and parents. They seek parents' perspectives by listening carefully and trying to understand parents' point of view and their feelings. EPPs use active listening skills rather than just blurting out the information and they really try to understand the feelings behind parents' decisions or actions. EPPs make time for conversations in which they focus on the moment, pace the conversation, and temper the information to the needs of the parent. They use language that is clear and direct, interpreting words or concepts unfamiliar to the parent, and clarifying or repeating information as necessary. They are truthful about next steps, about not knowing all the answers, and about the certainty of uncertainty. They are transparent and open to sharing, not to convince parents of one or another option but to explain to parents why they are talking about certain things so everything makes sense to the parents. EPPs find that *taking the time to explain things makes a difference.*

Sharing information in these ways is based on EPPs perceiving parents as part of the team caring for the child and they value parents' input. They recognize that parents *know better than anyone else what we might do, because you're the parent and you're the consistent person.* As a result, parents feel empowered by actively participating in their child's care. EPPs also encourage parents to contribute to making choices and decisions about the child's care. Further, EPPs both accept and support parents' decisions, even if the parent's decision differs from what providers might choose for themselves or their own child:

> I've had lots cases where the family is given two options—both very realistic and good choices—and the family chooses the one that I wouldn't do for my family. But I understand that and say it's not that they were choosing a bad choice but one of two viable options.

EPPs' broad worldview enables them to recognize that it is the parents, not PHCPs, who must live with the consequences of decisions.

Giving Bad News

Giving bad news is a particular type of sharing information and has the potential of empowering or greatly distressing parents. It stands out among PHCPs as a traumatic event for both parents who receive bad news and the PHCPs who deliver it. Many PHCPs perceive giving bad news as a dreaded event and hope for some practical advice about how to complete this procedure that would make it so much easier to do. Even though giving bad news is often thought of as a physician's responsibility, other PHCPs such as nurses and social workers also frequently are the bearers of bad news for parents. Bad news from physicians most often pertains to distressing diagnoses or poor prognoses, but nurses and social workers also engage in bad news conversations, for example, a nurse telling parents that their child is going to be moved to another location or a social worker conveying to parents that they are not eligible for a much-anticipated social service. In the parents' eyes, these conversations also are instances of bad news.

In fact, as described earlier, bad news for parents is any information about some change in the child's condition or treatment that disrupts the parents' sense of stability and triggers the shock and distress of the start of another transition. But for parents, though the news is often disturbing, how it is presented to them makes a significant difference. EPPs understand the importance of their approach to sharing bad news:

> I think it's natural that everybody pulls back from having to say something that you don't want to say that's difficult. You know it's going to have a big impact on the person you're speaking to, but the approach to what you're doing and the understanding of what you're doing, it seems to me to make all the difference.

EPPs perceive that any information, including bad news, is not simply something to be delivered to parents; instead, it is a reason to engage authentically with parents in conversation. At the core of this approach is the attitude that everyone is in this together. When viewed from the broader context of a conversation with parents, the giving of bad news retains its significance but lessens PHCPs' anxiety associated with giving or delivering such news because it becomes a conversation that is part of establishing or maintaining a relationship with parents. Parents then can also feel empowered rather than solely distressed. EPPs provide evidence that such interactions are possible and even feasible as a goal that all PHCPs can strive for.

Teaching

Teaching is an empowerment activity that occurs in response to parents' need to learn. It is not typically a one-time lesson; rather, teaching begins with the child's admission, continues throughout each hospital stay, and prepares parents for caring for the child at home if and when the child is discharged from the unit. When teaching, EPPs continually strive to find out from the parents what they already know, want to know, and/or feel they need to know. They consider whether parents are in need of instruction about how to do certain procedures, or if parents need guidance about what changes or symptoms to watch for in their child and what to do in response. As needed, EPPs provide teaching about how to manage the child's care at home, or what parents can expect in the current phase of the child's illness.

Children with CCCs may live with their condition for a long time, so their parents have much to learn, for example, about drugs, side effects, and what signs or symptoms to look for in their child. Parents in NICU often have learning needs about managing technology: *There are all sorts of things that the parents need to learn when babies go home with a trach, a home ventilator, overnight CPAP, home vent training, maybe CPR-type training, airway-type training.* EPPs implement strategies accordingly and with the aim of empowering parents. These families need a lot of education; so EPPs start teaching a new family as soon as they have a diagnosis. Teaching is then ongoing throughout the family's stay.

EPPs engage parents in learning by encouraging them to search beyond what EPPs teach them and some parents become *super experts*. Parents go on the internet, which allows some families who by nature would not necessarily be active participants in their child's care to get involved, and then they bring their suggestions and ideas to the PHCPs. EPPs encourage parents to embrace their learning and to become very active in their child's care. At the same time, continually exploring with parents what they have learned on their own is also an important aspect of teaching. Doing so alerts PHCPs to the need for clarifying or even correcting what parents know (or think they know) based on various resources they may have used, such as the internet or other parents:

> Parents come up with a suggestion and you just want to go, 'Oh, my God!' You have to start back-pedaling trying to say less, maybe spend a couple of sessions with them to try and get them off of what they saw online about something. So sometimes it's not helpful, all this stuff that they can read.

EPPs are particularly skilled at how they respond to some parents' unusual ideas:

> You can't just blow a family off and say, 'Oh, you know, acupuncture on the big toes has never been any good for a baby who can't feed or can't move!' You have to listen and acknowledge what they are saying. Just say, 'Well, you know, I'm not really sure but I can look and see.'

In teaching, EPPs take into account varying parent backgrounds, such as educational level, experience with illness or caregiving, and language spoken. Some families have no experience whatsoever with the diagnosis—they need to be taught everything so that they can learn to take care of things right away and be empowered. Specific parents need additional teaching:

> Parents who haven't finished school, and who have been essentially disempowered in life, aren't as empowered when they come into the health care system. So, we work really hard, because those parents, they

become experts too. Sometimes it just takes a little bit longer and you have to spend more time teaching them about the care of their child. But they all become experts. They all speak the lingo at the end of it.

EPPs' knowledge and experience make them aware of patterns that indicate what could happen and help them anticipate what a parent may need to know or do in the immediate or longer-term future. For example, when a baby has a scalp vein IV inserted overnight, it is helpful to anticipate the parents' responses to an unexpected change in their baby and choose to greet the parents upon their arrival in the morning to offer an explanation. An EPP's observations and knowledge of child development, parental coping with loss, and teaching/learning theory can help them to involve parents with their child and also prepare for their impending bereavement:

> I was troubled by parents who spent the whole time on their iPads and iPhones and their little girl just wanted some interaction. She would get it from staff, but then she would bond with us and we would leave at the end of the shift. So, she would feel the constant loss of being left and her attachments were in the wrong place. But she was so young and didn't know how to do anything differently. I realized that I had to redirect her attachments back to her parents and get them to come out from their iPads and iPhones. They were very young themselves, so they were just keeping in touch with their life and this was a huge thing that was going on for them. It was much easier to be in iPad-zone than to be faced with the reality of their beautiful child dying. And I can't blame them for that at all but redirecting her back to them was key. She would ask me to read her a story or to snuggle her and I would say, 'You know what, I would love to snuggle you but I can see that your mom really wants to have a snuggle with you. How about we get your mom to put down her iPad and come over here and give you a snuggle?' And so, I kept redoing and redoing that and it was quite amazing—eventually it started to change.

At the same time, some EPPs see a need for improvement in what is taught to parents and to the process of teaching as sometimes family teaching is not done early enough. They note, however, that in a busy environment, *It is sometimes easier for staff to do things rather than teach parents how to do the same thing*. These EPPs also acknowledged that a lack of knowledge among some of their colleagues seems to be one reason why teaching does not happen when it is needed. These EPPs described how they not only do their best to fill the gaps in parents' knowledge but also how they strive to teach their colleagues in a nonjudgmental way so that in future their colleagues will be better equipped to teach parents.

EPPs also demonstrate creativity in how they teach parents. For example, EPPs recognize that some parents like to cling to the hard facts and will bond with their child's monitor. So EPPs might introduce parents to a monitor by teaching them what the monitor is and how PHCPs know by the sounds what is happening. But they will also put their hand in front of the monitor and encourage parents to focus on their child instead of the monitor. EPPs also frequently teach by modeling or demonstrating, for example, when a mother is too frightened to touch her tiny baby:

> So I took her hands physically and washed her hands, and then asked her to put her hands on the side of the incubator. I went to the other side of the incubator and I drew her hands up and I put my hands on hers. So, the next time she visited, the next day, she didn't need me to do that. And she progressed to putting her hands inside the incubator and gently stroking her baby.

EPPs often find too that demonstrating is especially useful for teaching non-English-speaking parents about how to carry out technical skills, for example, tracheostomy care:

> I lay out all these things, so even though the mother might not understand English she can understand me pointing to something. Then she watches me and sees how I do it first. Then I hand it to her and, with a hand gesture, indicate, 'Now, you do it,' and she does it. And you go thumbs up if it's good.

In addition, EPPs frequently refer parents to printed materials and review such materials with them, word by word. They are also adept at using drawings, schematics, and videos, some of which they make themselves for parents.

In summary, unlike many PHCPs who tend to focus mostly on technical/clinical competency, EPPs engage in competent direct care activities within a context of interaction that also guides them to include empowering behaviors when they interact with parents.

Further Thoughts on Direct Care Activities

The common thread throughout direct care activities, whether *doing-for* or *empowering*, is that EPPs do everything with intention. They are purposeful and thoughtful in how they approach families and in how they determine the most appropriate course of action in collaboration with the parents. They have an awareness of where families are in their current transition and they work to align their care with families' needs. As they engage in interaction, EPPs consciously consider their intent for each interaction. They bring a mindful awareness of their own energy before starting an interaction and they are clear on their reasons for initiating interaction. Further, EPPs pay attention to the methods or processes they intend to use within an interaction to reach the outcomes they hope to achieve, but they also are mindful of what they learn from parents so that they can use that learning to help them truly meet the parents' needs. EPPs' ways of doing-for and empowering within direct care activities are most often reflective of how they engage in the process of attuning (see Chapter 4).

EPPs focus on what they are doing, though not to the exclusion of con-textual awareness as they understand that they may need to pause their current activity to attend to other priorities. Their focus is not just on com-pleting the task itself as they also focus on interacting with the parent while doing a task. EPPs realize that deliberately focusing on what they are doing differs from carrying out a procedure automatically; so they strive to be pre-sent for parents regardless of the reason for their interaction.

Another thread within direct care activities is that competency in techni-cal skills is essential for every PHCP. Therefore, EPPs recognize the impor-tance of obtaining, maintaining, and extending competency in doing-for skills. EPPs also value mentorship and both formal and informal supervision so that novice PHCPs as well as practicing clinicians can continue to build their skills and provide the best care possible for families. Continuing edu-cation in the clinical setting is viewed as a critical component of develop-ing technical skills and EPPs see clinical educators as important facilitators of skill development. Concomitantly, EPPs also value empowering activi-ties, and so they expect mentorship, supervision, and continuing education efforts to enhance PHCPs' abilities to engage in empowering activities.

Similar to many other aspects of our model, PHCPs can refine their direct care activities by learning from not only themselves but also from others. Asking questions of your own practice, observing how colleagues engage in direct care activities, and talking with others about both doing-for and empowering behaviors can all contribute to your development as a competent, caring clinician who values and engages in interaction with parents and others.

Considering Doing-For versus Empowering in Clinical Practice

You might find it easier to identify specific tasks or *doing-for* activities because, from your perspective, they seem in many ways to be more concrete than *empowering* activities. Doing-for activities also may be more familiar because your education and experience to date have emphasized such activities. But you may be surprised at how often a direct care activity can involve a combination of *doing-for* as well as *empowering* behaviors. For example, when changing a dressing (doing-for), you may also be teaching the parent how to do the dressing themself (empowering). Increasing your awareness of what types of direct care activities you are comfortable with, as well as how often you incorporate empowering into your practice, may help you to consciously choose ways of enhancing your interactions with children and parents.

One way to begin increasing your understanding about what you do and how you are in practice is to think about your to-do list from your last clinical shift. Identify what was on your list and then, for each item, consider if it was a *doing-for* or an *empowering* activity based on how we have described them in this chapter. Ask yourself the questions in Box 5.1. As you become familiar with the types of direct care activities normally involved in your practice, we encourage you to expand your repertoire and actively build on what you currently do so you can optimize your care of children and their families.

Considering Doing-For

Use the questions in Box 5.2 to help you learn how to meet the needs of parents as you contemplate thinking about what is important to parents, for example, competent practitioners who provide care at appropriate times. Consider how you prepare for *doing-for* activities. Observe your colleagues to see what they do with regard to doing-for activities—you can learn a lot by reflecting on how others engage with children and parents and by talking with your colleagues about your observations. Another area to reflect on is whether your focus during a doing-for activity is such that you inadvertently or deliberately exclude interacting with patients and their families. Sometimes, students and less experienced clinicians have difficulty paying attention to other people because they are so intent on safely completing a task. Yet, parents are clear that they at least want to be acknowledged, so think about your level of engagement during doing-for activities. You may believe that parents will only see you as a safe and competent provider if

---

Box 5.1: Direct Care Activities—Differentiating Doing-For versus Empowering: Questions for Consideration

- Identify what was on my to-do list from my last clinical shift. For each item, was it a doing-for or an empowering activity?
- Did I have difficulty determining into which category each item fell? If so, why do I think I was having difficulty?
- What proportion of the items was doing-for compared with empowering?
- Was the proportion what I anticipated?
- Or was I surprised at what activities were actually empowering rather than doing-for or were also empowering and not only doing-for?

Box 5.2: Direct Care Activities—Doing-For: Questions for Consideration

Preparing

- What do I take into account prior to starting a task?
- Do I gather all the items I need before I enter a patient's room?
- Do I give myself enough time to complete my task safely?
- Do I consider if I might need help for the activity and then alter my schedule as needed? Or do I push ahead regardless?
- Do I think about whether or not the timing I prefer is good for the patient and family?
- How flexible am I if I have decided on an appropriate time but the parent does not agree?
- Think about what I normally do if a parent asks me to come back later. Am I comfortable with how I typically react, or is there a different way I might engage so that the task gets done but the parent also feels heard?
- How often do I consider if a specific activity could also be used as a teaching moment for parents, so incorporating empowering into the activity?

Engagement

- Do I normally interact with a child and their parents while I am engaged in doing-for activities? Consider if I deliberately choose to exclude engagement.
- Am I intentional in engaging/not engaging or do I just do whatever I normally would do?
- How do I decide whether or not I am going to engage? Are there some situations more than others that guide me toward engaging? If so, what do they involve?
- How would I feel if I chose to actively engage with children and parents every time I performed a task?
- What do I think the outcome might be for children and parents if I always chose to actively engage? For myself?

Making Mistakes

- Do I think it is possible to be a competent practitioner yet also need help at times or perhaps make a mistake in my practice?
- How willing am I to ask for help? About what? From whom?

- What do I do if I make a mistake? Do I tell someone? If so, who? If not, then why not? What internal and external factors affect whether or not I take action if I make a mistake?
- Do I think that parents will not trust me if I make a mistake?
- How do I use my doing-for skills to engender parents' trust in me? What else do I do or say to parents to enable them to trust me?

they trust you and you do not make mistakes. But though parents do want competent caregivers for their children, they also recognize that errors can happen and they are willing to forgive someone who is honest, accepts responsibility, and strives to prevent similar mistakes in the future. They recognize that PHCPs are human beings and human beings are prone to making errors despite their best intentions, so consider how you handle making mistakes.

Considering Empowering

You need to think about what *empowering* means to you. See Box 5.3 for questions to help you with the various empowering activities. One aspect of empowering means including parents as part of the care team. Consider whether or not you treat parents as part of the team and if you help parents in *navigating* the system. Remember that parents in the neutral zone of transition typically feel lost and uncertain; it can be difficult to be with parents in this state but EPPs choose to be with them. Reflecting on what you have learned in this chapter about the importance of *supporting*, especially for parents in the neutral zone, consider how you work with families who are in transition. Offering support to parents is an empowering activity that is beneficial to both parents and staff even though it takes time and can add to workload. EPPs value making the time to support parents because they understand that supporting is very important to parents. They also are aware that when they are quietly supporting parents they may look to others as if they are not very busy. Rather than thinking that you do not have enough time, consider that both EPPs and parents refer to how significant connections occur within *meaningful moments*. You might then think about intentionally choosing how you are going to use your time and energy in moments of interaction, that is, you could decide to focus your attention on making a connection with the parent in the moment. Even little things, such as a smile in passing, a hello as you enter the room, or a touch on the arm during a procedure contribute a lot to exemplary practice. You might also consider how it is within moments that your body language, your facial

Box 5.3:   Direct Care Activities—Empowering: Questions for Consideration

- What does empowering mean to me?
- How does my definition fit with the description in this chapter?
- How do I think my definition affects the proportion of empowering activities I have on my to-do list?
- When observing colleagues, what makes me think that someone is performing empowering skills well? What do such colleagues do? Say? How do they act?
- What aspects of colleagues' behaviors might I emulate to enhance my own empowering skills?

Parents as Members of Team

- Do I regard parents as part of the care team?
- If I do, how do I involve parents in the care of their child? How do I involve them in making decisions about care?
- How do I know whether or not parents in my setting feel a part of the team?
- What have I seen colleagues do to help parents feel part of the team?

Navigating

- When a new family comes onto the unit, how do I help parents navigate the system? Or do I assume that someone else is carrying out the work of navigating?
- How often do I ask parents if they have questions about how things work or who people are? When do I share information about resources with parents?
- How do I learn where the resources are?
- What types of materials are available in my setting to orient parents to the health-care system?
- What else might I do within my professional role to navigate for parents?

Transition

- Think of a time when a family I worked with was in transition. How comfortable was I simply being with that family? How could I have better supported the family?

- Are there certain types of transitions that are harder for me, for example, when there is a new diagnosis or when a child is dying?
- How do I support parents who respond in anger to news about their child's condition?
- What do I do when a parent is crying?
- Am I someone who chooses to go to parents in these situations to support them in the ways that they need? Or do I ignore, dismiss, or mollify their concerns?

Supporting

- Do I worry that others might think I am not doing my work if I do not appear to be busy?
- What does being busy look like to me, and what does work mean to me? What makes me feel as if I look busy to others?
- Does work only include tasks, or are there other important aspects of work, for example, empowering parents, that are important to me?
- Am I aware of times when I portrayed a sense of busyness that interfered with my ability to offer support to parents?
- How do I think parents feel if they sense that I am too busy?
- How do I use meaningful moments to support parents?

Sharing Information

- How do I determine what information a parent needs?
- How do I typically share that information?
- How do I know that a parent has understood the information I have provided?
- Think of a colleague who I think is particularly good at sharing information with parents. What do they do that impresses me? How can I incorporate those behaviors into my own discussions with parents?
- What is it like for me to give bad news? Am I anxious about having to give bad news? Do I find myself eager just to get it over with?
- Do I think I can alter my anxiety by changing my perception from giving bad news to having a conversation to share the information?
- Consider how empowering it can be for parents when rather than just giving bad news EPPs share information in conversation. How can I have a dialogue with parents about bad news so that the parents feel empowered?

Teaching

- Think of the information that I typically teach to parents. What is it that I teach?
- How do I help parents learn when I am teaching?
- What approaches (e.g., drawings, props, diagrams) do I most commonly use?
- Do I have easy access to a stock supply of teaching materials that I can use to help me with my teaching? If not, what kinds of teaching aids would I find helpful in the teaching that I do?
- How can I obtain such aids? Who do I need to talk to?

expression, your tone of voice, your gestures, your eye contact, and so on all might contribute to making moments meaningful.

A main goal of *sharing information* is to make sure that parents are well-informed because being informed helps parents to feel empowered. But how do you know what information a parent needs, how to share that information, and if a parent has understood you? See Box 5.3 to help you with these questions and more, including how you might enhance your teaching of parents. Parents want the knowledge and skills necessary to independently care for their child. Therefore, *teaching* is a crucial empowering activity for all PHCPs to have in their toolbox. Some of the ideas that EPPs have shared would be useful for you to consider. You also might consider writing down what it is that you usually say—then read it over carefully and refine as necessary to improve it. Share your words with your colleagues and discuss together how to refine your language even more.

The direct care activities comprise the inner stabilizing band in our model of exemplary interaction. In Chapter 6, we discuss the outer stabilizing band that comprises eight connecting behaviors. These two components of the model function together to help keep the facets of attuning working smoothly.

Reference

Bridges, W., & Bridges, S. (2019). *Transitions: Making sense of life's changes* (40th anniversary ed.). Hachette Book Group.

6   Connecting Behaviors

> *I think sometimes you meet a parent and there is that quite instant rapport. You just con-*
> *nect and then it's easier going. But I can think of families where I meet them and I think,*
> *'I don't know how I'm going to connect with this parent,' and then it's almost like a very*
> *delicate, sensitive building, so not rushing it and not doing it all in one go. It's part of the*
> *process and it takes time.*

Just as a windmill needs multiple parts for it to work optimally, so too does exemplary interaction between parents of children with complex, chronic and potentially life-threatening conditions (CCCs) and their PHCPs. The outer stabilizing band of a windmill wheel helps keep all the blades connected to one another so that they function in unison. In this chapter, we discuss eight connecting behaviors, all of which are reflected by this singular outer stabilizing band. These behaviors permeate every aspect of interaction and build connections between PHCPs and parents. We found that each connecting behavior merges into the other connecting behaviors and, in fact, it is challenging to isolate them as separate or independent skills even though the literature is replete with articles and even books that address the need for skill in each of these behaviors as singular behaviors. We have learned that though skill in each is necessary, skill in all of the connecting behaviors is required for exemplary interaction. At the same time, such skills alone are not sufficient for PHCPs to optimally attune to the needs and concerns of parents. Connecting behaviors are only one important aspect of exemplary interaction.

As noted in Chapter 1, this study was inspired by parents identifying that it was the human quality that characterized excellent interactions with PHCPs. Our findings indicate that, arising from their commitment to authentic engagement, EPPs believe that *connection sits at the core of what it means to be human*. For EPPs then, the ultimate purpose of these connecting behaviors is to optimize the quality of EPP–parent interaction by connecting with parents on a human-to-human level to aid in determining and responding to what matters most to parents during each particular encounter. Connecting behaviors facilitate taking the other into account by

DOI: 10.4324/9780429352393-6

reaching across conventional role boundaries to see another in more truthful and responsive ways. Connecting behaviors are not accidental, nor do they occur by chance. Rather, connecting behaviors are guided by EPPs' intentional desire (commitment) to respond authentically to the sadness, suffering, challenges, uncertainties, and hopes experienced by parents of children with CCCs. EPPs interact with many parents over the course of each day and cannot be expected to reach the same level of connection with every parent. However, EPPs realize that with every encounter the parent's trust in PHCPs is enhanced or diminished, even if only by a degree, by the nature of the human connection between them. The eight connecting behaviors are: (1) *Empathizing*, (2) *Showing Kindness*, (3) *Suspending Judgment*, (4) *Building and Maintaining Trust*, (5) *Listening*, (6) *Pacing the Message*, (7) *Maintaining Hope*, and (8) *Staying Positive*.

Empathizing

Empathy has been defined in multiple ways and by various people. In a concept analysis of empathy, Patterson (2018, p. 219) proposed that the defining attributes of empathy are "cognitive understanding, affective understanding, and communication of understanding back to the individual." The antecedents of empathy, factors that must be present before empathy is possible, are "consciousness, cognitive functioning, caring capacity, and the ability to communicate," whereas the consequences or outcomes of empathy, are "perceiving that one's situation is understood by others (Reynolds & Scott, 1999), feeling respected (Wiseman, 1995) and cared for by another (Bailey, 1996)" (Patterson, 2018, p. 220). Empathy is a crucial component in the provision of quality care to patients and families and it is inextricably linked to the other connecting behaviors in our model.

EPPs differentiate empathy from sympathy: *With empathy, you are truly with someone and make a difference. Sympathy is saying 'I am sorry for your loss'*—an acknowledgment for another's distress but without feeling what they feel. At the core of EPPs' empathy is their desire to engage authentically with parents, to recognize the complexity of the parents' situation, and then to consider what they can learn from parents as a basis for devising the most appropriate response. Because EPPs value authentic engagement with parents, they are curious about individual parents' experiences and they understand that *narrative interaction is the best way to know what information parents need, what they want to know, how they make decisions—to know them.* By really listening to parents, EPPs grasp what the parents are feeling, can imagine what it might be like, and feel some of what parents are feeling, that is, they have empathy for the parents. They find it helpful to imagine what it might be like if they were in the parents' shoes because *I'd probably be just like those parents and that helps me to reserve judgment about parents' stressed-out behavior.*

EPPs, however, explicitly dismiss the common definition of empathy as walking in another person's shoes because they realize that it is impossible to do so:

> We must be good listeners, good learners, honest, and non-judgmental because we have no idea of what goes on behind families' closed doors. We don't want to pry into their personal lives; we respect their situation from the point of view of openness. We just need to listen to the story they tell so we are not jumping to conclusions based on assumptions.

Additionally, EPPs are aware that trying to put yourself in another's shoes runs the risk of *taking on* the feelings of others. EPPs strive to not take on parents' feelings nor let themselves become overwhelmed; otherwise, they would not be able to do their jobs. EPPs do not, for example, think about situations in this way: *I'm sitting there listening to the doctor give the mom some bad news, thinking, 'Oh my God, if that was me in her shoes or even in the doctor's shoes, I think I would have to leave the room. I don't know if I could do it'.* EPPs have learned that such reactions usually indicate a need for some self-exploration and learning. In this situation, the PHCP felt overwhelmed because of not differentiating the mother's or doctor's potential emotions or sensations from their own reactions. EPPs are not unmoved by others' emotions; rather, they are aware that empathy requires that they do not lose themselves in the process. They maintain their own feelings, their own center, and they remain grounded within themselves: *You have your own emotions, but you have to put them aside a little bit to do the job, but not so you become a stone.*

EPPs acknowledge that knowledge and experience help to broaden their perspective on parents' experiences and, as a result, increase their capacity for empathy. For example, memories of caring for a family member with dementia or cancer or having a child of their own who is disabled or has died, enabled these EPPs to extrapolate from their experiences to understand and empathize with parents of children with CCCs. EPPs emphasize that they do not typically share their own experiences with parents unless they sense that it might be helpful for the parent, for example, *I may tell some moms about my child's story as a way of affirming the parent's feelings of being in the hospital day in and day out, being exhausted, and how their world becomes very, very small.* Recognizing the challenges that parents face by being in the hospital or hospice also fosters empathy. EPPs understand that it is *hard enough for parents to deal with their own stuff, yet their stress is compounded by the settings where parents can hear and see what is happening with other families.*

When a PHCP is empathetic, then parents feel supported and cared for: *She's very empathetic, very supportive, cares about you and your family.* Understanding a parent's perspective even though it is different from your own is critical to empathy: *First, accept their feelings; don't challenge their feelings and don't deny their feelings. Just know that they are suffering and imagine how distressing that is for them and see how you can help them deal with those feelings.* Look beyond the superficial, for example, in a situation when a grieving parent is angry, reflect on this understanding so *you can see the pain before you see the behavior.* EPPs describe empathy as identifying with the human plight of parents:

> You are a better caregiver if you identify the parent as someone who is on the same journey that you are on. You are a fellow human being, a fellow traveler on the journey of life. This perspective engenders a type of respect that facilitates an understanding of the parent's lived experience.

Identifying with others' experiences involves connecting with people who are from cultures other than their own, though EPPs also acknowledge that parents are most likely to identify with other parents who are in similar situations because *they are walking the same journey* and, thus, EPPs encourage parents to meet and learn from one another.

Showing Kindness

EPPs referred to *kindness* as well as to *empathy,* so as two different concepts. Both result in parents feeling cared for, empowered, reassured, and/or comforted, but *showing kindness* is about enacting compassion and touching parents in a heartfelt way. Kindness involves a special moment that people remember. Kindness is evident when EPPs notice a need or desire in a parent and then respond in the moment by doing something for the parent that is out of the usual pattern of care, that is, different from what others have done or from what the PHCP themself might normally have done. It also is different from and more than being polite or following rules of etiquette. Showing kindness touches EPPs with a *heart surge* of warm and positive feelings, a deep sense of gratification. For example, while caring for an acutely ill baby, an EPP

> got the mom to gently wash her baby's eyes and his face. The baby died the next night and a message from the mom was passed on to me to say thanks because that was the only thing that mom ever did for her baby. That was very powerful for me.

Showing kindness does not necessarily take a long time, as for example when an EPP recognizes a parent seems tired and offers to make a cup of tea. However, the length of time depends on the particular act of kindness, and EPPs are willing to modify their scheduled plan of care or to stay beyond their shift to accommodate parents' needs—for example, the EPP who noticed that a mother was desperate to hold her dying child but realized there was no way to do it without help, so the EPP sat and held the tubes for three hours to let the mother hold her child and say good-bye.

Acts of kindness can range from little to large things. A father arrived at the hospice late at night after a long day of outdoor work and travel. He got up in the morning to find a breakfast of granola and yogurt. The cook, noticing the big, burly father and his disappointed expression, asked if anything on the buffet appealed to him. When dad said, *No, not really,* the cook then made him bacon and eggs. Dad said, *I'm a big guy but I started to cry. I didn't realize that I needed someone to look after me just a little bit.* The cook noticed, listened, and responded with kindness in the moment. Making a parent feel welcome is an act of kindness that all PHCPs can easily do and it can make a big difference to the parent. And, when parents experience an act of kindness, they generalize the resulting good feeling to other PHCPs and feel that *people here care not just because it is their job, but because they truly do care.*

Suspending Judgment

Being empathetic and showing kindness both require that PHCPs see others as human beings who deserve attention in a gentle way. Yet, *though it would be ideal if all PHCPs were nonjudgmental, we're not.* The human reality is that all people are influenced by their worldview and values, the lens through which they shape their assumptions, interpretations, and opinions. Everyone carries biases, for example, about race, gender, ethnicity, ways of behaving, height, or weight, which can lead to making assumptions about and then stereotyping others. Human beings tend to connect more easily with people they perceive as similar to themselves. For example, a vast body of research, as reviewed by Hall and colleagues (2015), indicates that health-care providers have implicit biases in terms of positive attitudes toward Whites and negative attitudes toward people of color. Suspending judgment then is especially important in situations where PHCPs perceive these kinds of difference between themselves and parents. Notably, EPPs are aware of this phenomenon and strive to bring attention to implicit biases at both personal and institutional levels. For PHCPs, however, assumptions often lead to judgments about what parents should and should not be, what they should or should not do, or whether they are coping well or not—but all according to the PHCP's own standards or measures.

One way that EPPs *suspend their judgments* of parents is to remember that it is not about them. Suspending judgment means not comparing the parent's situation to their life or personal experiences, that is, not thinking that *because you experienced something similar in your own life that it is applicable to this family.* Personal experiences, such as having a baby die, also have the potential of helping EPPs recognize the importance of suspending judgment because those memories can force them to examine their own previous judgmental behavior, for example, about the *drama* of grieving mothers. Having been on the other side of the fence, EPPs are able to understand that *you cannot assume anything about parents; instead, you need to find out from them.*

EPPs recognize the potential of their own expectations or opinions to influence the development of trust with parents of children with CCCs. This does not imply that EPPs ignore or deny their own assumptions or opinions; rather, they acknowledge them and intentionally suspend them so that their assumptions do not influence how they interact with parents. EPPs know that they all carry their own biases, but they work to understand what families are going through, for example, the grief of not having the perfect child, and they realize that families come with their own expectations and so PHCPs must put their opinions aside.

Building and Maintaining Trust

Trust is the basic foundation of any relationship and EPPs recognize that trust formation and maintenance are critical to their interactions with parents. Signifying that they too see trust as critical, nearly every parent talked about their need to have trust in the PHCPs who care for their child. For parents, trust means that they are confident the PHCPs will take good care of the child, which lessens parents' worries. Parents' trust is based on both the words and the actions of PHCPs—the authenticity of people's words is judged within the context of their actions; so PHCP behaviors are extremely important. Parents trust EPPs because they see EPPs as *competent, attentive to details, caring,* and *interested* in the child so they *do the right thing* for the child. Parents also appreciate that EPPs involve them, for example, by asking parents questions if the EPP is unsure about something, as well as hearing parents out.

EPPs are aware that credibility is a crucial factor in a trusting relationship with parents, and so they also know that their demonstrations of competency are vital in balancing those areas fraught with uncertainty. Because trust is a matter of obtaining credible information, parents must believe what PHCPs are telling them, but PHCPs too must believe the parents. When trust is present in a relationship, parents will be more receptive to hearing what PHCPs have to say and discussions, even about difficult topics or bad news, will tend to go more smoothly.

Recognizing that trust is not automatic and must be earned, EPPs realize that parents may initially experience distrust. Thus, from their first encounter with parents, EPPs aim to mitigate initial distrust by being competent and honest, thus creating *a safe feeling* that alleviates parents' anxiety and fear. If things do not go smoothly in that initial crucial period, then trust will have to be rebuilt or repaired, which can be time-consuming as well as a hindrance to the relationship. EPPs make time to talk with parents and through not necessarily long, but frequent encounters, EPPs let parents know they are *there for them*, which builds trust. Both building and maintaining trust are important for developing relationships because the cyclical process of parents and PHCPs getting to know one another builds layers of understanding that are then consolidated into trust. Any time a parent's trust is violated, interactions do not go well.

EPPs intentionally work to build and maintain trust by carefully *reading parents* and *making use of opportune moments so parents do not feel rushed or overpowered, taking things at the parents' pace*. For example, some EPPs often spend time in the vicinity of parents, paying attention to those opportune moments when parents might be ready to talk. They also see that continuity is a component of trust formation and maintenance; having the same person care for the child allows parents to see a familiar face and to develop a relationship with someone over a period of time. For EPPs, honesty and transparency are critical components of trust formation and maintenance; so they tell parents that they will have no hidden agendas, will be forthright with families, will not keep secrets from parents, and will admit when they are wrong. EPPs believe that being open and honest about their expertise and their limitations can gain and maintain parents' trust much more readily than PHCPs who claim to know everything and seem to be invulnerable.

EPPs believe that not knowing something is not a failure; rather, they believe that showing their vulnerability and admitting to not knowing *reflects your own humanness and makes you more relatable to parents*. For EPPs, being open about themselves, for example, sharing that they have two young children when a parent asks if they have a child or finding a common interest in baseball or the love of dogs, builds trust by allowing for familiarity. EPPs recognize that *parents really need to trust and realize that their PHCP is a human being*; EPPs believe that parents' tough decisions go better if they are familiar with who their PHCP is. However, EPPs are cognizant of being strategic as they strive to individualize the balance between involvement and distance. They ensure that they maintain the professional boundaries expected by the standards of their discipline while presenting themselves as fellow human beings.

A professional therapeutic relationship is dependent on trust and on keeping the patient/family at the center of the relationship. But at the same time, trust should be a mutually shared experience in which there is give and take on both sides. For parents, having PHCPs who work respectfully with them as partners is the difference between living in constant worry and being comfortable that their child is being well-looked after, despite how sick the child may be. EPPs are gratified when parents trust them and are willing to open themselves up to them.

Listening

EPPs perceive listening as a catalyst for promoting trust with parents: *When parents feel listened to, they feel a sense of connection, which leads to trust*. Many people assume that listening comes naturally, but parents often report a different picture: *It's nice to feel listened to because when you go to certain places, as a parent you don't feel listened to. And that's not a good thing.* It is important, therefore, to acknowledge that listening does not necessarily come easily to everyone or in every setting and that despite the extensive literature on listening and on how to develop listening skills, not every PHCP truly listens to parents.

EPPs understand and demonstrate that truly listening requires paying attention or attending to parents and to each family's story: *Attending to the words and the underlying levels of meaning, reading body language and facial expressions, observing what parents are not saying and watching their body language, their actions, and how that matches their words.* They show that not only are they listening to understand the other person but that they care to understand the other person. EPPs also indicate their readiness to listen by engaging in attending behaviors of physically placing themselves in a position that promotes interaction with parents. For example, depending on the structure of their particular clinical setting, they face the parent if standing, sit if the parent is sitting, lean in slightly, and make eye contact. But EPPs also are aware that eye contact is sometimes inappropriate, such as in some cultures where it is a sign of disrespect, or in an informal conversation when parents would see such behavior as awkward, and so they adjust their behavior accordingly.

Listening to a parent's story is respecting that parent's wish to be heard. Listening also leads to dialogue (a two-way process), which is needed in order to understand what really matters to parents in that moment so that EPPs can then design and take actions to help parents achieve their wishes. For EPPs, listening is an active, not passive, endeavor that is carried out carefully and with the intention to understand the parent, even if they disagree with what the parent is saying. EPPs validate parents' concerns that arise during conversation and they also verify their observations rather than making assumptions.

When PHCPs do not listen well, then parents struggle and become frustrated: *I'll try to talk to them and they'll say 'No, no, no' and they'll talk over me. But I'm asking a question—'Can I do that?' and they just choose not to listen, or they'll walk away.* Some parents refuse to have a PHCP take care of their child because the PHCP did not listen to the parents, lamenting that *I thought they were supposed to listen to you.* EPPs recognize that when parents do not feel heard, tensions increase and parents are dissatisfied. Therefore, EPPs make an effort to be fully present with parents. Presence is listening without interrupting, interpreting, judging, or minimizing and is especially important when people feel vulnerable, when life is particularly uncertain, and when it is hard to find meaning—just as it often is for parents of seriously ill children. EPPs demonstrate presence by being calm and by finding quiet times to talk with and listen to parents. EPPs note that really important conversations occur when parents can tell their story in those quiet times and often EPPs hear something they have not heard before. For some EPPs, the best time to listen is later in the night because the rush of the day is over; others carve out a time in their busy days that works for them and the parents.

EPPs often let parents take the lead in the conversation. They recognize that listening requires clarifying to be sure that they understand a parent's situation, while also verifying that the parent understands what they are saying. For EPPs, a good interaction is one where there has been honest communication about the realities, implications, and issues. Parents are then aware of the issues, have an understanding of them, and typically feel that they are an equal partner who has a voice. EPPs also strive to not react negatively to what parents say. They listen patiently and carefully to parents who disagree with the recommended treatment for the child and are adamant about trying an alternative treatment:

> I listened so much about how he wanted to treat his kid and then reviewed what he wanted to do. I actually had to go home and read about some of these really weird treatments. And, once I read about them, I went back to the father to say that I don't think this is going to work because of this or that. By listening to him—not just giving him lip service—by looking things up and explaining what would work and why, that dad actually did the full treatment as recommended. By just listening, you can get out of difficult situations and build trust.

As EPPs pay attention to each family's story, over time they come to see similar patterns emerging and this understanding facilitates even better listening skills and, thus, their ability to help appropriately. They make sure to use language and terminology that do not cause problems, that is, they talk at the parent's comfort level. EPPs also validate parents' concerns during a conversation, for example, reassuring them that there are no stupid questions or acknowledging emotion and reassuring parents that such feelings are expected among parents of a child with a CCC. For EPPs, not judging parents and trying to assist them as much as possible are basic to listening.

Pacing the Message

EPPs leverage awareness of the family's situation, gleaned from listening to each family's unique story, to determine the optimal pacing of message delivery. They are aware that families in crisis are likely unable to absorb large volumes of information, particularly when that information is complex, nuanced, and/or necessitates consequential decision-making. EPPs understand that if parents are distraught, then it is not a good idea to try to give them a lot of information.

To ensure that information is received in a way that families can understand and process, EPPs employ a variety of strategies based on their understanding of the family's needs and the child's current condition. Some EPPs use the first interaction as a way to establish rapport and a relationship with the family, focusing less on the details of the child's illness or the situation at hand and more on helping the family members know that they will be well-cared for by the health-care team. That first meeting is often used just to show parents that the EPP cares and is going to do their very best for the parents and their child. Other EPPs attempt to stage the conversation, starting with an overview and then, at a different time, progressing to the more specific details or to the decisions that the family will need to make. But if the general overview sinks in and the parents are ready, then the EPPs will give some more of the details at the initial meeting; otherwise, they come back later to talk. Still others use pictures or diagrams to help illustrate complex systems or processes and they may give parents notes the EPP makes about the discussion, which allows the family to revisit and further process the information shared.

EPPs have an awareness of the process by which families take in and absorb information, and they recognize the futility of forcing the conversation: *There's a rhythm and there's a time that is required for that change and that internalization to take place. You can wreck it if you don't accept that is the case or if you push too hard.* Additionally, they have awareness about the contextual factors that can impede parents' ability to fully engage in conversations, including financial challenges or the need for child care for other children in the family, and they take these factors into account when planning when and how to engage in dialogue with the family. EPPs know that if there are five children at home and the mother does not drive, then she will lie awake at night worrying and trying to figure out how to make everything work. An EPP assures the mother that they will find a way to make it work for her. EPPs also rely on their relationship with the family as they navigate particularly challenging conversations. When they have known a family for a long time, it is easier to have the conversation even when they are talking about things like death or a relapse, because they already understand how to interact with this family and the family has developed trust in the EPP.

The process of pacing the message is complicated when difficult information must be communicated immediately. In these situations, EPPs prioritize what information is shared and develop a plan for how and when to communicate the information they deem less critical, for example, *In the very first meeting, what's important is that they have a diagnosis and that they have hope that they can do it. The next day they need to know about the details.* EPPs stay attuned to the parent's emotional state and to the possibility of information overload, taking care to pause the conversation when a parent appears distraught or no longer seems to be processing the information that is being shared.

EPPs pace their message according to the parent's current goals and wishes for treatment, even when the goals may be different from those of the team. They invite the family into a dialogue and gently provide information that may impact how the parent thinks about their child's condition. For EPPs, *a dialogue is not a debate; it's about exchanging information and trying to learn and grow together with that information.* EPPs know that pacing of the message can be the mechanism by which families come to accept challenging information or make difficult decisions for their child, and they understand that these decisions can take time: *Maybe there isn't an answer today, but there may be an answer tomorrow.* [We must] *walk alongside them until they're able* to make their decisions. Finally, EPPs recognize that one of their roles in pacing the message is to help parents maintain hope.

Maintaining Hope

PHCPs are accustomed to conversations about hope. Parents of children diagnosed with serious, life-threatening illness normally start with hoping for a cure—and often until the very end of their child's life they hope for the miracle that will save their child. Some parents hope for remission, for a few more months of life, for their child's pain to be controlled, for their child to breathe more easily, for their child's suffering to end, for a peaceful death. But hope remains a mysterious and powerful force. EPPs see hope as part of the human condition; hopes are natural for everyone to envision. Indeed, this perspective has been evident throughout history, as evidenced by the Roman philosopher and statesman Cicero (106–43 BC): While there is life, there is hope.

At the core of what EPPs do to maintain hope is their commitment to seeking parents' perspectives to learn where they are with their hope. EPPs believe that you never take hope away from a family, and so they maintain hope as an integral aspect of how they engage with parents. They perceive hope as enabling, motivating, and sustaining for parents. Therefore, suspending judgment on parents' hope is essential to maintaining the parents' hope. Though EPPs recognize that some PHCPs think a family may have too much hope or that the hope is unrealistic, EPPs firmly believe that most parents do not want anyone to take their hope away from them. Parents noted the power of being given hope when getting bad news, despite understanding how sick their child was: *These health care providers did not paint a gloomy picture. They said, 'It's going to be really difficult' but there was always hope in what they told you.*

EPPs are aware that hope, like listening, is active, not passive, and that parents choose to hope in the face of terrible odds. They realize that if they tell parents *there is a 5% chance of their baby surviving then the parents will focus on their child being part of that 5%, not the 95% who die.* EPPs have reflected on the question of *Who am I to take away parents' hope?* and their answer is to *support the parents as they hope.* EPPs also recognize the dynamic nature of hope and how parents' hope changes as the child's condition changes. For example, *over time parents may no longer hope to see their newborn baby as an adult but may now hope to baptize their child before she dies.* EPPs acknowledge the emotional challenge of trying to help parents figure out what their hope is for or trying to help a family maintain some hope even when that hope is for something other than a long life. EPPs recognize and acknowledge the challenges and deal with them. For example, they use language that parents understand and that acknowledges the parents' hope, thus nurturing hope while also helping parents deal with rather than ignore or replace reality. Finally, because EPPs understand that information overload can contribute to hopelessness, they maintain hope for parents by giving them information in small doses and consciously, but cautiously, focusing on what matters to parents. They ensure that they have a plan to help keep parents grounded, reassured of support, and most of all hopeful because they know that without a plan, bad news sends parents off into a great unknown that is extremely difficult to manage.

EPPs also guard against giving false hope or false reassurance, what Florence Nightingale (1860, p. 54) called "chattering hopes," that only compound the sorrow parents must endure. Thus, EPPs are honest and realistic but also supportive of parents. Maintaining hope in the face of a child's devastating condition may seem pointless at best and gross malpractice at worst, but there are different ways of viewing hope. EPPs are familiar with hope from both a big picture perspective, for example, the possibility of the child surviving and thriving, and from a specific perspective, for example, a peaceful death. They embrace the concept of hoping for the best while preparing for the worst. They understand that miracles occasionally happen and that families need hope for the moment; parents cannot allow themselves to give up hope because that is what keeps them going every day. Indeed, this persevering aspect of hope fits well with the experience of parents of children with CCCs: *We're going to go on with this and we're going to have hope and that's how we get through our lives, plain and simple.*

Staying Positive

One of the reasons that EPPs stay positive is to sustain hope for parents, but they also have other rationale for staying positive. EPPs consciously choose to highlight the positives, no matter how small those aspects may be, so that they can balance out the negative and, thereby, offer support to the parents. For example, when sharing bad news with parents, EPPs also try to *bring up some things that are positive, that are going to help.* At the same time as they strive to stay positive, EPPs still recognize, not deny or cover up, the negative aspects of a situation. For example, when having conversations with a mother of twins, one of whom had died, an EPP would recognize that *the mom had sadness in her heart for the one who died* and they would talk about that child but also make sure to *end by also talking about the healthy baby.*

Recognizing the potentially negative impact on parents of the location of care also motivates EPPs to focus on the positive. For example, in a children's hospice

> when it is clear that the chemotherapy and the radiation are not working, that the child is there because he may die, I don't focus on that—I emphasize this is a place where you and your child can have time to rest as a family.

EPPs in NICU understand that NICU is not an inherently happy place because every infant has the potential of dying. They know that parents see tubes and monitors that drive parents crazy, so EPPs try to balance it all out by being positive and having extreme patience. When caring for distressed parents, EPPs focus on the positive because they realize that confrontational sentences only add to a parent's distress *so if you want to say something, make it good or don't say anything at all.*

EPPs seek parents' perspectives and involve them in making plans; they view making plans with parents as a top rapport-building skill. Thus, EPPs create conditions for parents to be actively engaged and to make decisions according to what is best for them in that moment, which parents see as positive and reassuring. Parents also appreciate EPPs who acknowledge that something has gone wrong and then try to find something good to come out of a bad situation rather than wallowing in the negatives. Sometimes, it is the parents themselves who set a positive tone, for example, making the most of every single moment of their child's short life, making life fun for the child and for everybody else on the unit too. A positive focus provides a kind of warmth, a way of staying human. It decreases parents' uncertainty for the immediate future and gives parents something to look forward to, which enables them to maintain a positive attitude.

For many parents, having a positive attitude is important in helping them deal with the stresses associated with their child's condition: *You have to at least try to see the positive in every day. It's easier to do at times, depending on the week, the day. I try to stay away from negativity, but having a positive attitude definitely helps.* Indeed, some parents tell other parents that the best advice they can give is for parents to stay positive. A positive attitude in PHCPs is also important to parents. Some parents even make a conscious effort to stay away from PHCPs who are grumpy, rude, or never smile, or who talk only about what is wrong. EPPs have a personal sense of optimism that enables a positive focus and that is observable by other PHCPs: *The excellent ones know how to find the happiness button. For some people, you can't find the happiness button, but if you can, then you are happy too.*

Further Thoughts on Connecting Behaviors

As we reflected on EPPs' connecting behaviors, we realized that those acts facilitate the creation of a bond with parents in which EPPs are entirely present with the parent. This ability to be present derives from EPPs being solidly grounded or centered within themselves. As a result, EPPs convey a sense of quietude that enables them to connect with parents on the parents' terms. EPPs are able to be silent while finding out what is most important to parents and then using their knowledge, skills, and expertise to attend to those concerns. EPPs clearly connect in ways that indicate the situation is not about them; they leave their egos at the door. They differentiate the type of judgment they are trained to exercise in their professional roles from their need to suspend judgment of parents. Doing so also requires that they suspend judgment of themselves and see themselves in the same light as they see parents: As unique, worthy, individual human beings. EPPs realize that they cannot be gentle in judging others without being gentle on themselves. They empathize with parents by holding their own emotions in mindful awareness rather than over-identifying with the parents' emotions. They are sincerely hopeful and optimistic without giving false hope to parents. They are aware of their own limitations and strive to continue to learn and grow. They present with a calm rather than harried manner and notice opportune moments for showing kindness. By conveying their clear intention to stick with parents through the challenges of caring for a child with a CCC, EPPs hold open a space within which they and parents connect in a trusting and meaningful way.

The concept of holding space is not unique to our findings. In fact, this concept is seen in the counseling field as an effective therapeutic skill. Holding space is a conscious act of being present, open, accepting, and protective of what another person needs in the moment. It is broadly used to define the act of being there for another. It means to be there physically, for example, with a hug or a gentle touch on the arm, and also to be there non-physically, for example, by offering your complete and full attention without the need to respond, interrupt, or comment. Those who hold space for others are self-aware, compassionate, and without judgment—characteristics common to EPPs. Though people often assume otherwise, engaging in connecting acts or holding space does not come naturally to many people. Such skills must be learned and practiced.

Considering Connecting Behaviors

To enhance further learning about your own skill in connecting behaviors, or in holding space, you might consider reflecting on the questions in Boxes 6.1–6.3 in relation to each of the connecting behaviors.

As with other aspects of our model, PHCPs can learn from themselves as well as from others as they develop and enhance their connecting behaviors. There are many questions that you might ponder as you think about your own practice and the practice of others, especially when observing and reflecting on those colleagues who are adept at connecting behaviors. When you consider *empathizing*, start with reflecting on what differences you see, if any, between empathy and sympathy so that you have an understanding of your own perspective (see Box 6.1). In relation to *showing kindness*, you might consider if you are someone who is known for showing kindness. Given that *suspending judgment* may not come naturally to you since a person's personal assumptions, biases, stereotypes, or expectations can affect their ability to connect with parents and others, consider how you might

Box 6.1: Connecting Behaviors—Empathizing, Showing Kindness, Suspending Judgment: Questions for Consideration

Empathizing

- What differences do I see, if any, between empathy and sympathy?
- Do I express empathy to others? If so, then in what ways?
- Are my behaviors and words similar to those of colleagues I would consider to be EPPs? If so, in what way? If not, then what can I learn from EPPs to help me further develop my own empathy skills?
- How do I express sympathy to others? How do my sympathetic actions differ from how I show empathy?
- Whether I think empathy and sympathy are the same or different, are there resources I might access, such as books, that could help me be as clear as possible about what empathizing means to me?
- Remembering a time when I felt overwhelmed with emotion, what happened in my life to trigger that emotion?
- What, if anything, have I done to help me manage feelings of being emotionally overwhelmed in my own practice?
- Do I choose to engage in emotional situations or do I find excuses to absent myself?

Showing Kindness

- Am I known as someone who shows kindness to others?
- Do I have a memory of someone showing kindness that can still bring me joy or perhaps tears to my eyes? Was I the one showing kindness, or was it someone else? What happened in that situation?
- How might I incorporate awareness about acts of kindness into my own practice?
- Do I pay attention to the little things?
- Do I feel that I am too busy to include acts of kindness in my practice?

Suspending Judgment

- Am I aware of my opinions and judgments?
- How easy is it for me to suspend my judgments or opinions of others?

- How do I put aside my opinions and judgments?
- Am I drawn to certain types of parents more than to others?
- Am I more comfortable with people who are more like me?
- What do I do when I am faced with a parent who causes me to feel some form of discomfort?
- Am I willing to have a close friend from any culture or religious group? From another political party?
- As I walk down the street, do I engage with a homeless person as another human being?
- What is my attitude about a person who is obese? Has a cognitive disability? Has a physical handicap? Who smokes? Has a different sexual orientation from me?
- What do my responses tell me about myself?
- What might be the source of my biases?
- What behavior(s) do I think represent an ideal parent of a child with a CCC? How do my expectations affect my interactions with parents who do not meet my ideal?
- What colleagues do I consider as being able to work with anybody, regardless of race, ethnicity, religion, and so on? How do such colleagues act? Do I act in a similar manner?

increase your awareness of your own opinions and judgments. Think about the relevant questions in Box 6.1 and how your answers may affect your ability to suspend judgment of parents.

Building and maintaining trust requires that you develop a relationship with parents and that you engage in two-way dialogue. Think about your own goals regarding building and maintaining trust and reflect on what you could do differently to help you develop the kind of relationships that EPPs have with parents (see Box 6.2). *Listening* is of great importance when trying to understand parents, and parents value feeling listened to. But true listening is not something that comes naturally to everyone. Use the appropriate questions in Box 6.2 to think about how you listen and ways in which you might improve your listening skills. Giving appropriate attention to *pacing the message* can feel like a challenge in the midst of a busy shift, yet consideration of pacing may be the key to helping families understand, process, and act upon information important to their child's care. As you think about your ability to effectively pace the messaging for families, you might start by considering how and at what pace you yourself best receive information from others (see Box 6.2).

Box 6.2: Connecting Behaviors—Trust, Listening, Pacing the Message: Questions for Consideration

Building and Maintaining Trust

- Thinking of a time when I needed the help of another PHCP, what were my expectations of that PHCP? Did the PHCP live up to my expectations? Why? Why not? What did they do or say?
- What do I think an ideal PHCP should be?
- Do I meet my own expectations?
- Thinking of a time when I felt vulnerable, what response from another person did I find helpful? Unhelpful?
- What behaviors in another person demonstrate trustworthiness to me? Are these behaviors ones that I demonstrate in my own practice?
- Have I had an experience where someone violated my trust? Or I violated theirs? What have I learned from those experiences about developing and maintaining trust with parents?
- How do I view my own level of competence?
- Do I think parents perceive my competence as credible?
- How comfortable am I in being open in my conversations with parents?
- What do my professional guidelines say about being open with parents? Do those guidelines fit with what I believe about openness?

Listening

- What was it like for me during and after an interaction where I truly listened? What was it like for the person I listened to?
- What does it mean to me to be present?
- How good am I at listening or being present?
- What helps me to focus on what the other person is saying?
- Does my mind wander to other tasks awaiting my attention?
- What is my usual body posture, for example, relaxed or rushed?
- Do I usually prefer to stand or to sit when talking with someone?
- During conversation, how comfortable am I with direct eye contact?
- What is my natural tendency when there is silence in a conversation?
- What is my internal response when the person I am talking to is preoccupied? Or angry? What do my responses mean for me as a PHCP?

Pacing the Message

- How and at what pace do I best receive information from others?
- What happens when I receive too much information too quickly?
- How do I know how much information a parent can handle?
- What strategies do I employ to ensure that parents are getting the right information at the right time?
- Thinking about a time when I recognized that a parent had become overwhelmed with information, how did I help to support them?
- How do I engage parents in dialogue about their child's condition, particularly when there are difficult decisions to be made?

Box 6.3: Connecting Behaviors—Maintaining Hope, Staying Positive: Questions for Consideration

Maintaining Hope

- What do I get most hopeful about?
- How do I maintain hope in my own life?
- Do I think that hope should always be maintained in my personal life? In my own practice?
- How do I respond when another's hope seems unrealistic to me?
- If I have refused to maintain a parent's hope, how did it make me feel? How did the parent respond?

Staying Positive

- Do I see myself as a positive person? In what ways?
- Do others see me as a positive person?
- What do I think is the source of my positivity or negativity?
- What is the difference between staying positive and being a Pollyanna (someone who has irrepressible optimism and tends to find good in anything)?
- Do I think that staying positive is always necessary in my personal life? In my own practice?
- Under what circumstances would I not want to stay positive in my personal life? In my own practice?
- How do I respond when to me another person seems to be unrealistically positive?
- If I have refused to be positive when talking with a parent, how did it make me feel? How did the parent respond?

As we discussed, EPPs and parents value *maintaining hope*. Reflecting on your own approach to and attitudes about maintaining hope can help you to help yourself as well as parents. Finally, *staying positive* is another important connecting behavior. Ask yourself the questions in Box 6.3 to help you consider how to enhance these connecting behaviors in your own practice.

When you are finished with this chapter, go back and review our model in Figure 2.2. You will see that so far we have discussed the upper part of the model: Worldview, values, and commitment, attuning, direct care activities, and, in this chapter, connecting behaviors. Now we turn our attention to the legs of the model, to the supports that hold up the upper parts of a windmill. In the next chapter, we will discuss the personal factors that provide a solid foundation for the components of our model as discussed so far.

References

Hall, W. J., Chapman, M. V., Lee, K. M., Merino, Y. M., Thomas, T. W., Payne, B. K., & Eng, E. (2015). Implicit racial/ethnic bias among health care professionals and its influence on health care outcomes: A systematic review. *American Journal of Public Health, 105*(12), e60–e76. https://doi.org/10.2105/AJPH.2015.302903

Nightingale, F. (1860). *Notes on nursing: What it is, and what it is not.* D. Appleton and Company. http://digital.library.upenn.edu/women/nightingale/nursing/nursing.html

Patterson, J. (2018). Empathy: A concept analysis. *International Journal for Human Caring, 22*(4), 217–223. https://doi.org/10.20467/1091-5710.22.4.217

7 Personal Influencing Factors

Flexibility is a component of going against your inclination and trying something different. In other words, don't do the same thing with everyone, and don't assume that what you did before will work again every time. The health-care provider must be open and have a sense of curiosity about what would happen if trying a new approach. Self-awareness is needed for health-care providers to know their own style. Knowledge is needed about what other approaches might be tried.

In order for a windmill's windwheel mechanism (the rudder, hub, blades, and connecting rings) to work properly, the windmill must have strong and sturdy legs. Each leg has to be as strong and steady as the others. The legs are further stabilized by struts that connect the legs to one another. Similarly, EPPs' personal factors provide a solid foundation that supports the development and evolution of their worldview/values and commitment to authentic engagement and enables them to carry out the blades of interaction. For EPPs, the stability of the legs, the four personal factors—*Knowledge, Self-awareness, Flexibility/Open-mindedness,* and *Curiosity*—is enhanced by two struts—*Self-care* and *Past Experience* (clinical and maturational learning).

Knowledge

EPPs demonstrate an expansive disciplinary knowledge base about the scientific and technical aspects of their discipline, obtained through their profession's educational curricula and their subsequent practical experience. They understand that part of professionalism is having both the knowledge base and the capabilities they are supposed to have in their respective roles. EPPs recognize that their accumulation of knowledge and expertise is a process and a responsibility; thus, they perceive ongoing professional development as a requirement in order to keep up with the ever-expanding knowledge in their field: *As someone who is supposed to have the best knowledge in the field, then I should always update myself so I have a good understanding of the latest cutting-edge technology.* Therefore, EPPs seek to continually expand their disciplinary knowledge by participating in various courses, workshops,

DOI: 10.4324/9780429352393-7

and other types of special training that allow for certification or membership in professional organizations. They recognize that attending conferences is an excellent way to learn; regardless of discipline, they recommend that all PHCPs start attending conferences early in their career. EPPs also seek to learn about other health-care disciplines so that they may work collaboratively with their colleagues.

Such disciplinary knowledge is a priceless gift and is mandatory for exemplary practice. EPPs and parents alike highly value and respect this knowledge. However, many traditional educational programs in health care typically focus on teaching facts, critical thinking, and logical problem-solving. This learning focus yields knowledge and confidence that facilitate being in charge during critical situations, but, at some points, factual knowledge reaches its limit and that is when PHCPs may feel lost, uneasy, and carried beyond what they *know in their heads*. For example, PHCPs may not know how to connect with parents who are different from themselves in some way or know *how to answer the desperate questions of distraught parents about their child's prognosis*. In such situations, EPPs demonstrate another type of knowledge that stems from their keen interest in the breadth and depth of human experience. This interest is reflected, first, in their extensive general knowledge about an array of topics—for example, art, music, sports, and pets—that facilitates EPPs' ease in conversation with parents and others, including their colleagues, who are from a wide range of backgrounds. Second, their interest in human experience, as reflected in their worldview/values and commitment to authentic engagement, is expressed in their extensive social/emotional knowledge. It was this type of knowledge that parents noted when describing excellence in interactions:

> She was so knowledgeable but when we were doing the dressing changes together, she didn't come in as the expert and this is the way it is; she came in as somebody who genuinely cared and was invested in the support that we had. She guided me but she also let me take the lead in doing those dressing changes.

This type of knowledge is the link that facilitates connecting with other human beings, getting to know them as persons, and understanding what individuals are experiencing. In moments of shared unknowing, a magical moment of connection shows that being human is much more important than being fully in the know. This type of knowledge is akin to Goleman's (1995) concept of emotional intelligence (EI). EI is the ability to recognize, understand, and manage your own emotions and to recognize, understand, and influence the emotions of others. Simply put, EI means both being aware that emotions can drive your behavior and affect other people (positively and negatively) and learning how to manage those emotions—your own and that of others—especially when under pressure. For better or for worse, individuals' appraisals of every personal encounter and their responses to those appraisals are shaped not just by their rational judgments or their personal history (including their social, cultural, and spiritual influencers) but also by their emotions. Human beings have two different kinds of intelligence—rational and emotional. Both kinds of intelligence are required for decision-making, but emotions can have an impact on someone's ability to think critically—or rationally—about a situation at hand. Conversely, emotions can also assist with decision-making; they can help guide an individual toward or away from a particular course of action. Neuroscientists posit that feelings/emotions are typically indispensable for rational decisions. Moreover, an individual's emotional learning through life experiences sends signals that streamline their decisions by eliminating some options and highlighting others. Those with strong EI recognize this connection between the rational and the emotional and use it to manage their interactions with others.

Connecting with others in meaningful ways incorporates ethical behavior and is more than simply knowing the rules and regulations for conduct related to a PHCP's particular discipline. The ability to engage in ethical relationships with others begins with self-knowledge, which is an ongoing, evolving process that requires PHCPs to make a commitment to knowing the truth about themselves. For example, EPPs recognize how they have changed over time. They understand that instead of everything being either right or wrong—according to what they consider is right or wrong—there are usually shades of gray in any given situation and that the clear-cut and easy-to-find solution tends to mean they have not yet examined all of the possibilities. Therefore, EPPs' knowledge is tempered by ever-present uncertainty and ambiguity. Basic to EPPs' self-knowledge is the realization that their decisions require them to pay attention to mind, body, and emotions.

EPPs are fascinated by and committed to human-to-human interactions. They perceive that the accumulation of this type of knowledge and expertise is a meaningful and lifelong process. Typically, PHCPs attend to keeping current and up to date with disciplinary knowledge and research, and also even with general knowledge. But in addition, EPPs seek knowledge about themselves. They are aware of and understand their own capabilities, character, feelings, and motivations, and they are willing to express that awareness to others honestly and appropriately. Self-knowledge is attained through self-awareness.

Self-Awareness

Self-awareness is the conscious knowledge of one's own character, feelings, motives, and desires. For EPPs, being self-aware means constant reflection on what a situation or interaction is doing to them internally as well as to others. They look for triggers for their own and other people's reactions as they seek to understand how they affect others and how others respond to them. Being cognizant of their impact on other people and conscientiously sensitive to how others respond to them, they adjust their behavior accordingly to deal with others positively. They choose different words or emphasize different things depending on the family and what is happening. EPPs assess situations moment by moment, day by day, so that they can understand what is evolving. They contemplate how they are changing through interaction and realize that who they are today is at least a little different from the day before.

EPPs express interest in learning more about themselves as a way to enhance their interactions. In describing the components of attuning in Chapter 4, we discussed how reflecting and self-awareness are closely interrelated. EPPs understand that they cannot just focus on who they have met with that day and what the parents' issues are. They realize that they bring their whole selves, their past experiences, and their opinions on life and people to interactions. Therefore, they know that they must be aware of all they bring and make themselves consciously think about it so that they can engage with parents as optimally as possible. EPPs believe that being self-aware of the challenges in their own lives, including what currently influences or threatens them, gives them insight that makes a difference to their ability to be sensitive, patient, and perceptive when helping parents.

Some EPPs engage in reflection by keeping a journal or at least writing down or audio-recording their thoughts and feelings on a regular basis, preferably daily. Such actions can *capture the mood of the moment* and help EPPs understand the number and range of emotions they have experienced and what they have learned from them. When EPPs, through reflection, identify something lacking in themselves or something they could have done better, they seek to learn more; they want to change so as to optimally enhance their practice. EPPs note that they often discover new things about themselves by reflecting on their reactions or responses to new environments, clinical situations, people, or demands where they face new challenges. Some EPPs facilitate the development of self-awareness by reflecting on their personal history and the extent to which they think that past experiences have affected their current experiences. They also consider their various roles in life—for example, as nurses, physicians, social workers, as clinicians, teachers, or researchers, as parents or grandparents, as aunts or uncles—and contemplate how they affect and are affected by those roles. Some EPPs seek counseling or spiritual guidance in a serious attempt to more deeply know and understand themselves.

EPPs seek to accurately judge their own behavior and to recognize and respond appropriately to others during their interactions with parents and other people. They are especially mindful of the importance of self-awareness in caring for parents of seriously ill children. They realize that PHCPs whose own needs need to be filled fail to establish good boundaries and struggle in this work. They have learned that they should not spend time with these families while hoping that families are going to fulfill their own unconscious needs; families cannot fulfill those needs and PHCPs should not expect them to do so. Unlike some PHCPs who are less aware and whose need to be needed is so profound that they choose an area that does not fit, EPPs understand their own unconscious drive to do this kind of work. This understanding brings a certain groundedness that helps parents in the chaos of a child's death, the most ungrounding, catastrophic experience imaginable for many people.

Engaging in the process of developing self-awareness takes courage, and sometimes EPPs admit to not liking what they see in themselves. One area that may pose challenges is when parents are *difficult, the ones that aren't necessarily nice and are quite obnoxious*. EPPs understand that there are difficult people in all aspects of life, so it is not surprising that some parents are also difficult. But it can be a struggle for EPPs to stand back and not judge these parents for how they behave:

> That's a tricky one, that's something that I think you constantly need to work on, because no matter how much we say we're nonjudgmental, we all have our own histories, our own upbringings, and our own stuff on board and it can be hard at times.

Moreover, it is difficult to be objective when thinking about one's own perceptions. What PHCPs think parents see may be quite different from what parents see:

> It was my first experience with this doctor. She was being very, 'Well, I know what I'm talking about and you don't. I'm the doctor here.' And she said, 'I want to do this, this, and this because I have a feeling that something is going on.' I asked if she'd talked to Dr Smith. She said, 'I am the oncologist on call, I do not have to talk to Dr Smith about it.' I responded, 'Well, you are not Sarah's oncologist, you are the oncologist on call and I would really prefer if you ran it by Dr. Smith first.' She was really snarky with me from that point on. She didn't tell me that she had access to test results that I did not know about. She wouldn't say what she was thinking even when I asked if she could give me more than 'You have a feeling.' She said, 'No, I just have a lot of experience.' Explain that to me. Don't tell me you've got a 'feeling.' It's not good enough for me. I've never seen you before in my life and you're making life decisions about my child. She was not very nice, really unprofessional in her tone and attitude. I don't think she has any awareness of the fact that that's not a nice way to talk to parents.

As a result of their self-awareness, EPPs are cognizant of internal thoughts, feelings, and reactions while interacting with others. They tune into their own feelings, as well as to the behaviors and feelings of other people, which in turn contributes to EPPs knowing more about and having a better understanding of themselves. EPPs work at sorting through what they can do as individuals, and they strive to set realistic expectations for themselves and for parents about what can be done and what the EPP can or cannot do. Self-awareness promotes honesty and sincerity as well as flexibility and openness so that EPPs are not afraid to be—and to be seen as—caring human beings.

Flexibility/Open-Mindedness

EPPs convey an attitude of flexibility and openness; they *take things as they come, whatever the day or an encounter might hold.* Being open allows for flexibility in how EPPs respond to and adapt to changing situations, helping them prioritize and be creative so that they can carry out their work in new ways. Flexibility also means operating on the parents' timeline rather than the EPP's: *You let parents take their time; they're in charge of their child.* Open-mindedness means that EPPs intentionally open their minds to new ideas and new ways of thinking. They *think outside of the box* and are willing to consider varying points of view. Further, they are adamant that openness is required for their approach to interacting with parents as fellow human beings and because of their belief in parents' capacity for doing what is right for themselves and for their child, they think that *parents make the best decisions they can, and you have to believe people are coming from a good place.*

Open-mindedness is integral to eliciting parents' input and to dealing with families on their terms while attempting to understand the whole range of issues that are affecting the child and family. Flexibility is relevant to how EPPs and parents negotiate the child's care, in determining what the EPPs will do and what the parents will do. This negotiation is a matter of give and take, of partnering in the care. Flexibility also implies taking a tailored or individual approach rather than a one-size-fits-all way of doing things. It is a component of going against their inclination and trying something different. In other words, as advised in the introductory quote to this chapter, *Don't do the same thing with everyone and don't assume that what you did before will work again every time.*

EPPs are open to considering what parents suggest, whether or not they actually believe the suggestion might work. If EPPs think a proposed suggestion is not viable or might cause harm, their flexibility leads them to investigate the parents' suggestion and then bring information back for further discussion with the parents. Being flexible means that rather than judging parents, EPPs respect the parents' decisions even if the EPP disagrees with a decision: *If a parent says, 'Well, I'd like to be there if CPR is necessary, I want to be there,' I am willing to think about that or at least be open to engaging in conversation about it.* Flexibility and open-mindedness mean giving up some control, something that some EPPs do easily as they contrast flexibility with rigidity, Type A behavior, or an inability to deviate from strict routine or a set way of doing things. For EPPs, these terms imply that concentrating on the more technical doing-for activities can lead to rigidly following routines and adhering to patterns that limit their ability to respond effectively to parents. EPPs have developed the skill of being flexible while maintaining order in what needs to be done. These notes made by a research assistant in our study after observing a family meeting provide an example of a positive difference in outcome when a lack of flexibility is replaced with flexibility:

> The general tone of the health care providers was one of 'This is what we are going to do.' It seemed that if there were questions, or stalling, or some hesitancy from the parents, it almost felt like, 'Oh now, you have messed up our plans!' There was no flexibility and people were getting frustrated. The mother exclaimed, 'What about this testing? Are we looking into this?' One physician did not dismiss the mother's questions and calmly said, 'You know, that's a good question and something we can consider.' So even though Dr. Singh didn't say 'Yes, okay, we'll do that tomorrow' and she had her own reservations, she showed some flexibility. It totally diffused the stress and the defensiveness because the parents were really trying to make their point and nobody had been open to listening.

Flexibility and open-mindedness can be particularly important when a child is dying. Setting aside procedures and routines in order to give parents some moments they will never have again is something that EPPs are aware of. Openness is especially critical when having difficult or challenging conversations with parents:

> When parents realize that you're actually willing to open this difficult conversation and that you're not pushing for an answer, when we say, 'We want you to know that we're open to continuing this conversation in the most supportive way we can,' it has a paradoxical effect of opening the conversation.

EPPs' flexibility reflects their ability to slow down, to portray a sense of calm, and to be willing to adapt to a situation as it changes. Their capacity for open-mindedness allows them to sit with uncertainty, to wait and see, and to be open to hope.

Flexibility and open-mindedness also allow EPPs to recognize the needs of parents and change priorities in the moment. What might initially seem to be the most important thing to do may not be the case in a given situation:

> I think being rigid about schedules is just kind of dumb. If you need to give a medication at 2pm, you can give it within half an hour, especially if it's working with the family schedule. If a mom is going to cuddle until 2.15, just hang the med when you put the baby back in the incubator rather than stop the cuddle just to start the medication.

For this nurse at that point in time, family bonding time was more important than a 15-minute delay in beginning a medication.

Being flexible and open can contribute to EPPs' successful reflection because as they reflect on a conversation with a parent, they can *literally hear things or see things differently than you did at the time because you're open to the question of 'Was there something more happening there than you're aware of?'*

Being flexible and open is not always easy even for EPPs:

> The hardest thing for me is flexibility. For example, if you go into a room with preconceived ideas about what you are going to do and the parents come up with something else, then it's like, 'Oh, I didn't prepare for something else; what do I do now?' So, you always have to go into a room with the idea of this is an open slate. You may have ideas of what you want to say, but it can totally change from what you expected. You have to change direction, and you have to say 'Okay, how am I positioning myself now so that I can go ahead?'

Even though flexible and open-minded EPPs are sometimes challenged, their self-awareness helps keep them on track. They realize, for example, that if their mindset puts people into categories, then it will limit their ability to actually be open to others in a way that would be helpful. Therefore, they constantly check in with themselves to catch such issues early.

Flexibility and open-mindedness in adapting to their work assignment can also be challenging for EPPs. Fluctuations in workload demands are common in health care, and flexibility is needed as schedules and situations change. One way of thinking about flexibility is to consider how you interact effectively and in a way that does not feel as if you are distracted or already in the next situation. Interacting with someone while reading text messages, answering phones, or speaking with others outside of the current conversation is detrimental to an interaction, but these are things that happen all the time. The skill of being flexible and still maintaining order in what needs to be done is a component of exemplary interaction and a skill that EPPs are able to master, often by practicing mindfulness. This issue of PHCPs juggling multiple demands on their time was one of our fundamental research questions: "Why do some PHCPs with the same demands on their time interact more effectively than others?" We found that EPPs provided answers to that question.

An important aspect of EPPs' knowledge is to know their strengths and limitations and to accept what they know and what they do not know. Such knowledge requires self-awareness which, in turn, contributes to being flexible and open. An aspect of admitting one's limitations requires humility and a desire to address those limitations. Being willing to explore, to learn, and to know stems from curiosity.

Curiosity

From the time they are students in postsecondary educational programs, PHCPs are bombarded with facts and socialized into thinking that knowledge, competence, and certainty are the authoritative hallmarks of health care. Such expectations also greet them as practitioners in health-care settings where the expectation is to practice with certainty. Pediatric health care is, however, an uncertain practice. One only needs to look to the experiences of parents of children with complex, chronic and potentially life-threatening conditions (CCCs) and the variation in outcomes for these families to validate this uncertainty. We identified that not only is uncertainty an inherent and normal aspect of the work that PHCPs do every day but also being curious is an essential capacity for EPPs and supports them in dealing with uncertainty. Some EPPs remember being a novice and experiencing anxiety, for example, clammy hands and increased heart rate, because of the fear of not knowing. But as they became more experienced or followed the advice of mentors to *trust your knowledge, trust your curiosity, you have the tools—go for it!* they learned to work within uncertainty.

Curiosity is the propensity to seek out new information and experiences; it includes an intrinsic interest in learning and developing your knowledge. Researchers have shown that being an open, curious person is linked to healthy social outcomes and a wide range of adaptive behaviors, including tolerance of anxiety and uncertainty, positive emotional expressiveness, initiation of humor and playfulness, unconventional thinking, and a nondefensive, noncritical attitude (Kashdan et al., 2013). Such attributes apply to EPPs, and, indeed, curiosity is a mindset for EPPs. They are curious about themselves and what motivates their feelings and behaviors, about other people and what makes them who and what they are, and about the way the world works. Curiosity requires EPPs to be open to seeing, hearing, and feeling what another person is saying or doing.

Curiosity also gives EPPs clues as to what to do next. For example, instead of asking How am I going to do this? they calmly ask, How am I going to do this? For EPPs, being curious is about being interested, inquisitive, and open to the uncertainty that is inherent in parents' experience of having a child with a CCC. EPPs want to know how things work, how they can make things work better, how they can determine a correct diagnosis and best treat it, why a parent may have reacted in a particular way, and why they themselves responded the way they did in a particular interaction. The personal commitment and curiosity that encourages them to try to understand what makes parents act in the ways they do also makes EPPs *patient enough and have the stick-to-it-ness* to work through all the elements to get to a place where they can make a difference. *Compassionate curiosity* is nonjudgmental. EPPs are curious about the parents' place of strength, recognizing that it may be very different from something they can identify with. They believe that if they create a safe place of nonjudgment and are sincerely curious, then people pick up on that sincerity and that openness and desire to really understand the other person. So rather than accepting something as inevitable or unchangeable, EPPs intentionally seek to learn more about how to better meet parents' needs; they keep trying within their means to *find the common thread to find out what's going on.*

Though curiosity is often spontaneous, sometimes it takes time and effort, especially when something is out of the EPP's area of expertise:

> When they say there's a feeding issue, the baby aspirates—I always ask, 'Can you educate me? What does that mean? What does that mean for the future? How are we going to get this baby home? How are we telling the mom? What word are we going to use to explain it? What do we have to offer with this problem?' So, gaining knowledge through curiosity in a highly medicalized environment when I'm 'only' a social worker takes a considerable amount of energy.

The curiosity of many EPPs is often palpable and evident in their excitement about what they have learned. They find their curiosity intrinsically rewarding and memories of their feelings of excitement, for example, when they studied for a certification, fuel their drive to keep learning more. Curiosity is also the source of some EPPs' energetic approach to their work:

> Curiosity—I love that! I want to be knowing that there are new things to learn and I can learn every day. And I do learn every day. If I wasn't curious, I wouldn't want to put out that extra effort. I think that's the difference for me. When I lose my curiosity, I know I'm starting to burn out.

Similarly, curiosity comes into play when EPPs sense that something is out of order or ask, *What is going on here?* Asking such a question actually can take EPPs outside of their comfort zone because it has to do with increasing, not removing, uncertainty. Further, their curiosity helps EPPs do the best they can despite how difficult a particular parent may be:

> Sometimes the people that we're working so hard to care for are just plain difficult people. Or they're in a place that makes them grouchy or like a porcupine or irritable. It's hard to carry through. In these situations, I've often been helped by a little phrase that I picked up 20 or 30 years ago: 'If you don't love somebody, you just don't know them well enough.' To me, that phrase links in with curiosity. If somebody is really difficult and you don't love them at all, it leads me to ask myself the question, 'What is it? Why is it that? Why is this person like this? What's been going on in their life? What have they been coping with?' And the curiosity pulls me forward in spite of the barriers, so it's helpful.

Self-Care

Care is often noted as a positive feature of human relationships, particularly in health care. A core value of any health-care profession is caregiving, that is, providing a caring response to a patient's plight. But the focus on caring for others is so deeply rooted in professional formation that the care of oneself is often overlooked and, in fact, often leads to PHCPs believing they are immune to needing care themselves. Yet self-care, one of two struts in our windmill model, is part and parcel of good caregiving for others. Commonly, the term refers to activities outside of work that strengthen individuals so that they can better cope with work stress. In all our settings, EPPs openly acknowledged the stress and strain associated with the nature of their work and they identified self-care as a top priority. They believed that they could not properly care for others if they had not taken the time to care for themselves. For EPPs, self-care is about more than focusing on their physical health; it is about being aware of their emotions, bodily sensations, and behaviors and needing to act in some way to protect their own well-being in all aspects of their lives, both outside and inside their workplace: *You have to care for your own body, mind, and spirit to do this work.* Self-care is essential to maintaining an EPP's personal integrity, that is, being able to maintain positive feelings of self-worth and self-esteem and to maintain energy levels, all of which provide the inspiration to carry on and are integral to exemplary interactions with parents and others (Davies & Oberle, 1990; Widger et al., 2009). EPPs reach their full potential as professionals and human beings when they practice good self-care.

To fulfill their commitment to remain present and fully engaged with their work and interactions with parents and others, EPPs are acutely aware of their need for self-care and, thus, intentionally plan activities to take care of themselves. EPPs believe that caring for their physical body is essential in order to care well for others; so they endeavor to maintain a healthy diet, get enough sleep, and engage in physical activity. Some enjoy activities such as hobbies or volunteering that offer respite from the daily stressors of working and living. EPPs find it helpful to share experiences with colleagues and to socialize with friends away from work. In addition, EPPs often acknowledge their need to disconnect or disengage for short periods of time in order to regain a sense of balance, particularly emotionally, and may take time for journaling or engaging in spiritual practices. Meditating or engaging in mindfulness practices is a common strategy for the rebalancing that helps EPPs focus on the present.

Some EPPs also seek help beyond the more common activities because although they can talk to their colleagues, sometimes they need someone from outside to point out that they seem to be struggling with an issue. The wrong help can be problematic: *I went to two counselors. The first counselor told me I needed to go on meds and quit my job, so I didn't go back to that one.* But the right therapist can be very useful: *I found one who is just able to listen and really brainstorm about 'How can we make things better?' and 'How can we make it so you can cope better?'* EPPs maintain balance between their work and personal lives but also acknowledge that these two integrated parts of themselves cannot be totally separated, especially when the meaning they find in their work overlaps with the meaning they find in their personal lives.

EPPs emphasize that self-care also requires another type of balance: Between socializing with others and having time to themselves for self-reflection. Socializing with others for leisure and relaxation activities is essential for self-care, but solitary time is equally important to EPPs. Solitude connotes being alone but not lonely; it conveys the sense of choosing to be alone. Solitude is a form of self-respect for EPPs that results from self-awareness and acknowledgment of the fact that they do not always respond to others when they want or need to be alone:

> I'm a believer in the practice that if you're not, for whatever reason, feeling like you can go there or devote the time, you don't get into it. So, for example, if I go for lunch and I'm feeling like I can't talk to anyone at the moment then I go sit by myself. I used to feel guilty about it and then I talked to one of my colleagues who said, 'No, actually that's more therapeutic.' And so, I think, for me anyway, I'm very conscious of knowing when there's moments that I need what I call my time-outs. When I know I can't engage in a particularly helpful way with someone then I just don't go there, because it's not helpful for anyone.

EPPs realize when they have reached their limit and need to step back from a situation, but they also caution that there is a difference between stepping back to avoid a situation and stepping back to reflect on a situation. Solitude is a time for an EPP to be with only themself, not with others, and to engage in reflections and activities that can better prepare them for interactions with others. EPPs often are active in seeking their solitude; they find walking, biking, reading, or other solitary activities a time for reflection: *I look forward to my early morning run through the park because it's 30 minutes I have all to myself before the emails, meetings, patients inevitability creep in.*

EPPs who commute to and from work take advantage of their time in the car or on public transit for solitary self-care. The journey to work is often used to reflect on their time at home and to prepare themselves for what they might expect at work, whereas traveling home allows time for reflection, for processing, and for winding down. That journey from work to home is very important for some EPPs, especially if they are feeling a little burnt out, because it provides a transition period and grounds them.

A major source of work stress for PHCPs was the fact that the children they care for are potentially or actually facing death. EPPs are highly aware of their need to acknowledge and accept their own grief reactions as particularly important for integrated functioning; so self-care also means that EPPs do not ignore or run away from death. Sometimes, though, they do remove themselves from the bedside of a dying child for 10–15 minutes so that they can regroup before coming back. A lot of sadness comes from having developed a relationship with the family, and then *when they leave* us—when their child's body leaves, and the parents go, and you know you're not going to see them anymore—it's this strange feeling that you have to face and deal with. On such days, an EPP might take a longer route driving home to reflect on the day to bring forward some fond memories of the family. EPPs note that caring for these children enhances their own awareness of death and, as a result, they can be open with the children and their parents in discussions about prognosis and attend to what really matters in the moment.

EPPs also understand the importance to their self-care of acknowledging and managing the emotions of grieving. They know that part of self-care is being able to not only show their emotions but also manage them so their emotions do not consume them to the point where they cannot function. EPPs realize that having the self-awareness to know what triggers them, being honest with themselves and others, and sharing their sorrow are all part of the self-care everyone needs to do:

> When I'm emotional and tearful about a child or parent, I need to think about that after. 'What is the trigger? Is there something else going on for me that has made me identify with this family in a different way? Is that an okay thing to do or do I need to step back a bit?' So, I think it isn't just about having tears, it's about thinking afterward about your interactions with the families and thinking about them before you go in again. That's good self-care and good care for the family.

EPPs recognize the value of the emotions that can result from caring for these children. They know that to deal with their emotions they need to listen to their body and what they are feeling. EPPs understand that if you go home after a day during which a child suffered a lot and you do not feel anything, then you should not work there anymore because you cannot be numb and do this work. But if you go home sobbing, then maybe you need to recognize that you have reached your limit for right now and need to step away from the situation for a day or two. EPPs commonly note that one way to look after themselves in sad situations is to *celebrate life despite the suffering and death that I witness*.

Valuing themselves through self-care is of utmost importance to EPPs' ability to preserve integrity. Cues and reinforcements for self-care come from both internal and external sources. An internal source comes from within the EPP: *Sometimes you have to have that self-awareness and that helps you do something about the situation that ends up in self-care.* Being able to laugh at themselves (facilitated by seeing a wider picture) as opposed to having a critical eye on the particular behavior that they perceive as wrong is also an internal source that supports self-care. Another internal way EPPs support self-care is to change their perspective, for example, if a situation is frustrating, then they choose to think or act differently. For example, an EPP who is having difficulty with a colleague might decide to go to work one day with a different attitude because they know that their choice might result in a good day. Reality checks during the day about what they have accomplished also are forms of self-care.

External sources of self-care include evaluation by management, peers, or colleagues and positive feedback from parents. Even on days when EPPs feel emotionally drained, hearing positive feedback is very helpful. They then feel good about themselves, for example, for supporting a parent or making somebody comfortable. EPPs also express gratitude for support from their own family members and friends who guide them through self-care. Further, mentors can be helpful in sharing strategies for self-care:

> Don't focus on what 'he said, she said.' It's simply how they're coping. It's nothing to do with us. It's not personal, so ride above it. Keep taking care of the baby, keep being consistent, and if you feel too much pressure, call somebody to support you; don't start getting into power issues. It's not about them. Everybody crashes in bad times and you see their worst; nobody is going to stay happy if their kid is dying. Why should we expect them to be normal and happy and have a good conversation with us? They're going to have some very frictional conversations. They may not even remember it when they leave—what they said, what they did—because it's a phase. It's how you think about the situation—it's learnable. But then you have to learn it in your daily life too—you don't just use it here. That's when it becomes second nature. When you use it outside in your own world, and you don't let things bother you, then they won't bother you here.

Other helpful mentorship advice focuses on disregarding the media because media often promote a negative sense of how the world works, for example, through showcasing vanity, jealousy, fighting, and power struggles. Instead, mentors advise EPPs to widen their knowledge by attending to other areas, for example, spiritual, educational, or self-growth endeavors, or to expand their altruism and help other people by volunteering. EEPs have learned that *You will get what you look for, so choose empowering activities and then you can use them in both your personal life and your work.*

Past Experience

In an ongoing process that supports the four personal factors, EPPs actively incorporate their learning from past clinical and personal experiences into their current practice. Consistent with their worldview and values, as well as how they strive for authentic engagement with parents, EPPs use their learning from their clinical experiences and their own personal maturation as a human being in their efforts to provide optimal care. Not only are EPPs aware of their ability to gain from different ways of learning, including learning-by-doing (clinical learning), but they also reflect on those experiences and can describe them clearly to someone else (aspects of matu-rational learning).

Clinical Learning

PHCPs frequently refer to the value of their experience, that is, the accu-mulation of actual experiences in their chosen field. Experience or practice is about learning to do what other members of one's chosen profession do and gaining proficiency in those skills: *There is a clinical part of learning—you learn to identify changes, you know more about what may be happening, you become comfortable with what you do.* Clinical learning may occur by noticing how the more senior clinicians do something; so you find out what works or not. Watching others do a procedure, for example, starting an IV, and identifying each step can provide encouragement that you too can successfully complete the procedure. By practicing their clinical skills—by *doing it hundreds and hundreds of times*—PHCPs become increasingly confident and competent. When PHCPs spoke about how they developed certain skills and how they learned to be more effective and competent in their work, they tended to associate their clinical learning with external rather than internal evaluation of their performance.

As PHCPs gain more experiences, clinical learning can also contribute to increased competence in their interactions with parents. They can come to understand that interaction is a skill they must learn, and learn to do very well. Over time, PHCPs can gain some skills and insights on how to interact with parents: *A doctor may give bad news hundreds of times and not feel good about it a single time. But after working out some of the bugs, they get practiced at saying it well with compassion and within a relationship.* It is important, however, to understand that though the competencies developed through clinical learn-ing are necessary for a PHCP to become an EPP, they are insufficient by themselves.

Maturational Learning

Despite their clinical experience, accumulated competence in clinical skills, and their increased comfort with interactions, not all PHCPs are able to demonstrate exemplary interactions with others because *a person has to learn from experience and also grow from it.* This perspective implies that another type of learning is required—something that we call maturational learn-ing. Maturational learning involves a process of attaining maximal clinical, intellectual, and emotional development. Such learning is not necessarily equated with chronology, nor with years of clinical experience; some of the older PHCPs did not demonstrate the results of maturational learning, whereas some younger PHCPs did.

Some EPPs identify the accelerated personal growth that comes from working with children who have CCCs and how they are learning from varied encounters with every family in the *university of life*. EPPs acknowledge that the lessons families teach them daily, sometimes hourly, or even by the minute, contribute to making them who they are. They also refer to the impact of the reverse, that is, of their personal lives on their interactions at work: *You evolve as a professional. Any of the life skills you learn in your life come back to your work. A person's personal life affects their development as a person.*

For EPPs, maturational learning is a more personal type of learning that occurs through reflecting on the meaning of their work in relation to their personal life goals. It results when EPPs become more aware of the interconnectedness of the professional and personal aspects of their life. This learning is fueled by acknowledging that the children they care for may die, and many children do. The value EPPs place on the connection between personal life goals and professional work with children with CCCs and their parents is profound:

> One of my life goals is to become a more awake, aware human being and this setting is certainly a playground in which to work on that. I think one has to work on that to do this work. It's learning about who I am and everything that means, so it's my own growth—that's a big goal and within that are the things that we experience here, that we witness, that are at the level of the big questions in life, the meaning of awe and of wonder. And I suppose it's almost more philosophical. 'What is death? What is happening there?' So not just to the child, but to the family and then to us as caregivers. 'What is happening for us?'

Further, awareness of the interconnectedness of the personal and professional aspects of their lives reinforces EPPs' worldview and the value of human-to-human interactions:

> When I reflect on what has made my work so fulfilling over the years, I mean I've changed through all my interactions. Seeing what I've seen and just being here through the ups and downs with so many families has changed me as a person. But what I find the most fulfilling and satisfying is that I've come to the place where I meet human to human— and we're all human. We support people of all these different world religions and worldviews and perspectives. At the end of the day we're all human beings and we're on this journey together.

Further Thoughts on Personal Influencing Factors

Reflecting on the personal factors that influence you can help you identify ways to enhance your professional practice and best support the patients and families you provide care for. As an example, you likely already try to stay on top of *knowledge* in your discipline, but how do you prefer to receive this new knowledge? You might consider some of the alternate ways of gaining new knowledge that we have discussed in this chapter. Also, see Box 7.1 for questions to get you thinking. Consider too how your general knowledge of the world and your *past experiences* facilitate interactions you have with others. Perhaps you have an interest in basketball and you use your knowledge of the sport to start a conversation with a parent who is watching a game on TV. Or maybe you make a connection with a patient or parent who loves dogs as much as you do. You might even use that information to distract a nervous child during a procedure or to take a parent's mind off worries about pending test results. These behaviors would be considered examples of EI, so reading the patient or parent's emotional state and responding in a way that supports and/or calms the situation. Reflect on the EI questions in Box 7.1 to help you increase your self-awareness of how you show up in your work with families.

Becoming *self-aware* is a lifelong journey that requires commitment, perseverance, and time. It also helps to be able to laugh at yourself. The first and foremost step in this journey is making a conscious intention to be aware of your own thoughts, feelings, emotional and physical responses, and insights into various situations. You then need to use critical reflection to learn from this awareness so you can better understand yourself which, in turn, will help you be more open to understanding others. EPPs increase their self-awareness by spending time reflecting on who they are and who they want to be, as well as how they can become who they want to be. Some EPPs find journaling to be a helpful aid in enhancing self-awareness. Journaling can be done in multiple ways, from a hand-written record in a notebook, to typed in a computer file, to tape-recorded audio files (smart phones make it easy to record your thoughts and ideas in the moment). Regardless of how you choose to record your reflections, reflecting and keeping a record of how you sort out your values, deal with difficult situations, or interpret events around you can all facilitate self-awareness. Self-awareness can help you build a healthy self-concept and strong emotional intelligence, as well as help you to identify and accept your strengths and limitations. The more you are aware of yourself, the more likely it is that you will be able to interact with others in an authentic and natural way. Self-awareness can also be facilitated by thinking about your personal background. Use the relevant questions in Box 7.1 to facilitate your reflections on self-awareness.

Consider how people expand their *open-mindedness* (see Box 7.2). One way is to purposefully open their minds to alternative ways of thinking about life and about their work. EPPs are *curious* not just about their external world but also about themselves. Some ideas you might consider regarding your own level of curiosity include: What thoughts, feelings, and behaviors arouse your curiosity? You also might consider past experiences when you showed *curiosity*. See Box 7.2 for relevant questions about curiosity and then think about a time you asked a question in a class. What was the response you received from the teacher? Were you commended for asking the question? Or was your question dismissed in a way that was embarrassing for

Box 7.1: Personal Factors—Knowledge, Emotional Intelligence, Self-Awareness: Questions for Consideration

Knowledge

- How do I prefer to receive new knowledge?
- How do I share new knowledge with my colleagues?
- How do I learn from others?
- Is there something in my own clinical area that I could initiate to help facilitate sharing of knowledge?

Emotional Intelligence

- When thinking of a colleague I believe consistently demonstrates EI, what do I see them do to combine their clinical expertise (garnered through clinical learning) and their life experiences (maturational learning) to care for patients and families?
- What makes me think that their interactions with patients, families, and their coworkers stand out?
- Do I use any of their strategies with patients and families?
- How can I learn to use some of the strategies that my colleagues use?
- When thinking about how the strategies I use have evolved as I have grown from my work experiences, what lessons have I learned from my encounters with those I care for? What personal insights have I gained?
- How can I share my strategies with others?

Self-Awareness

- Do I ever stop to think about the feelings and thoughts that arise in me as I care for patients and families or interact with colleagues?
- Am I sincere about not covering up my imperfections?
- Am I compassionate with myself?
- If I make an error, what do I do?
- How do I think about myself? For example, do I accept myself for who and what I am, or do I fight against who or what I think I am?
- Do I criticize or scold myself when I do not adhere to certain standards and values?
- When I do not know something, how do I then think or feel about myself?

- A significant way to enhance self-awareness is to pay attention to my body and to my emotions. For example, if I become aware that I am holding my breath in certain situations, what thoughts are being triggered for me?
- When I think about my life in general, is it filled with joy or weighed down with deep fears, anger, or sadness? What about when I am at work? Is there someone I could discuss these feelings with?

Past Experiences Affecting Self-Awareness

- How was I raised?
- How have my family and friends influenced the decisions I have made thus far?
- To what extent do my past experiences affect my current experiences?
- As I think about my various roles, how do I see myself in relation to the other people in my life?

you? Did you perhaps feel that you were never going to ask any more questions of this teacher even if it had been another student who had asked the question? What some people do not realize is that their response affects everyone who hears such an interaction. Further, others' responses when you or someone else is curious can either positively or negatively affect your willingness to continue to be curious.

No doubt you have heard teachers or speakers at the conclusion of a lecture ask: Do you have any questions? Depending on their tone of voice, facial expression, or body position, you likely got a clear sense that their question could be interpreted as: You don't have any questions, do you? Or worse, as: You'd better not have any questions for me! Often, it seems that teachers or other people in authority tend to have a preference for how people should answer a question. Think of a recent interaction where you asked a question of a parent or a colleague. Reflect on how you worded your question, as well as your tone of voice. If you are truly curious, then you will be curious about what the other person really thinks. Upon reflection, you might realize that you need to consider changing the question a bit. For example, rather than asking: Do you have any questions? you might ask a more open-ended question, for example, What questions (or ideas) do you have? Or better yet: I would be interested in knowing what you think about what I have said, or I would like to hear about your ideas.

Perhaps you have shared our experience of noting that when individuals think they know something, they are less likely to see what they do not know and, thereby, are less likely to learn. Such people lack the curiosity that is the impetus for learning. Given the propensity in health care to seek certainty, it may be a challenge but consider how you can adopt an attitude of being not quite so certain. One way might be to confront what you do not know. For example, perhaps you could intentionally put yourself in situations where you are experiencing new things. And perhaps you could make a habit of asking: What is interesting about this situation? About this person? About this parent? What is still unknown?

When people feel overloaded with information and perceive that they have little time, it is difficult to explore outside of the box. In such situations, PHCPs tend to rely on what they know and on the protocols or procedures they have been taught. Unless they have also been taught to pause, take a breath, and regroup, it is unlikely that their mind is open to dealing with uncertainty. But it is at this very point that EPPs pause, create a bit of space within themselves, and are mindful of their curiosity as a gentle reminder to look a bit closer, to learn a bit more about a parent's unique story that may be vital to their care. Remember that uncertainty and curiosity go hand in hand and may sometimes feel uncomfortable. At such times, you might listen to the messages from your body and use them as subtle hints to become more curious, slow down, and probe further. Keep in mind that when you are fully engaged in the act of reading a novel or watching a movie, you are okay with the fact that you do not know how the story is going to turn out. In fact, it is the not-knowing that sustains someone's interest in the story.

Self-care involves identifying what is important to you and findings ways in your everyday choices to meet your own needs. Self-care requires that you choose among your priorities, which can be challenging or even burdensome. Self-awareness about your bodily sensations, your emotions, and your thoughts is needed; reflection then helps to identify the actions required to ensure your well-being (see Box 7.2). So, as you go about your work, pause for a moment to think about what you are feeling at that moment (anxious, joyful, confused, worried, fearful?). What physical sensations do you have (sweating, holding your breath, a racing heartbeat)? What is going on in your mind at that moment (worrying about the time, your next patient)? When you have a few moments, or maybe at the end of your day, think about what is significant about this experience. How did you respond to what was going on inside yourself? Did you ignore the sensations or perhaps tell yourself that you were being silly? What might be a more compassionate response to yourself? Repeat the exercise at other times and respond with care to yourself.

Reflection is a compelling aspect of professional practice and is something that is most often done alone. Like other skills, it requires practice and one way to practice is to make sure you have times of solitude, even if you are

Box 7.2:   Personal Factors—Flexibility/Open-Mindedness, Curiosity, Self-Care: Questions for Consideration

Flexibility/Open-Mindedness

- How do I show my flexibility when working with families?
- Do I purposefully open my mind to alternative ways of thinking about life and about my work?
- In new situations or when looking at new information, do I keep an open mind, or do I assume that I know how everything works?

Curiosity

- What thoughts, feelings, and behaviors arouse my curiosity?
- How might I explore these aspects of myself, for example, by drawing attention to my inner experience?
- What captures my attention as I go about my work? What do I find pleasing or bothersome, interesting or irritating, happy or sad?
- Am I asking questions in a way that shows I am sincerely interested?
- Do I use open-ended questions or closed ones?
- Do I wonder about what is new in a situation? About what is still unknown?
- Do I consider what more I can learn?

Past Experiences Showing Curiosity

- As a child or adolescent, did my parent(s) scold or commend me for asking questions about how things worked or about other people?
- What was the response to my expressed wishes or desire to do things or go places? To my explorations around my home, in my neighborhood, and beyond?

Self-Care

- How aware am I about my bodily sensations, emotions, and thoughts?
- Do I respond to or ignore what is happening inside myself?
- Am I tired? Am I too sure of myself? Not sure enough? Am I in a hurry? Am I focusing on this moment?
- How might I set aside time and a place for quiet reflection (solitude) on a regular basis?
- What do I do to take care of myself?
- How do I show compassion to myself?

an extroverted person. Solitude is a resource for self-care. Consider taking notes on your reflections or keeping a log of your solitary activities. Keep in mind that many self-care activities depend upon you taking time for yourself.

When you remember a time that you forgot to fulfill a promise to a parent, or when you say: I could have done better or I could have given more of myself, you have to forgive yourself for being human. But you also must remember that you cannot pour water from an empty pitcher. To care for others, or to be compassionate with others, requires that you are compassionate with yourself when you experience your own suffering. You must keep current with yourself. You must be self-aware—which does not mean being engrossed or absorbed with oneself. Self-awareness will help you to acknowledge yourself, your strengths, and your limitations. Self-care will help you respond to what becomes clear to you in your self-awareness. Attending to your own experiences is a form of self-care because by doing so, you are caring for your own well-being.

As you have been reading the book so far, we hope you have kept in mind that just like a water-pumping windmill, our model of exemplary interaction cannot function without the wind to engage the process. In our model, the family is that wind and the relationships developed with families are extremely important. In Chapter 8, we will discuss professional relationships and maintaining boundaries between PHCPs and parents.

References

Davies, B., & Oberle, K. (1990). Dimensions of the supportive role of the nurse in palliative care. *Oncology Nursing Forum, 17*(1), 87–94.

Goleman, D. (1995). *Emotional intelligence: Why it can matter more than IQ.* Bantam Books.

Kashdan, T. B., Sherman, R. A., Yarbro, J., & Funder, D. C. (2013). How are curious people viewed and how do they behave in social situations? From the perspectives of self, friends, parents, and unacquainted observers. *Journal of Personality, 81*(2), 142–154. https://doi.org/10.1111/j.1467-6494.2012.00796.x

Widger, K., Steele, R., Davies, B., & Oberle, K. (2009). Exploring the supportive care model as a framework for pediatric palliative care. *Journal of Hospice and Palliative Nursing, 11*(4), 209–216. https://doi.org/10.1097/NJH.0b013e3181aada87

8 Pediatric Health-Care Provider–Parent Relationship

I do a lot of teasing and play with small children. The medical residents think I'm kind of silly, but it's completely deliberate. I build trust and I know I'm gaining not only the confidence of the child—when the child laughs with me, the parents relax with me. They know that their child trusts me and then that helps to create a relationship.

The importance of relationship is widely noted in the health-care literature. Patients and providers both state that a strong patient–provider relationship is key to achieving a high-quality health-care experience (Council of Accountable Physician Practices, 2017). But what exactly is the nature of a strong relationship? Sociologist Arthur Frank (2004), as a patient newly diagnosed with cancer, used an example from his care to provide an answer. He told the story of how a technician came to draw blood. As she went about her work, Frank commented on how skillful she was compared to some other technicians who had come to draw blood. She responded by giving Frank helpful advice on when and how he had the right to refuse access to his body. After she concluded with: "Remember, everyone who touches you affects your healing," Frank realized "That technician is the one who drew me into a relation of care—because care can only be a relationship, a dialogue not only of words but of touch" (Frank, 2004, p. 17). She was not only drawing blood as part of a diagnostic procedure, she was also affecting who he was as a person.

Similarly, the ways in which EPPs touch human beings who are in distress are central to the relationships they form as PHCPs. Their words and actions stem from their worldview and core values and are expressed in their ability to form meaningful bonds with parents.

In a windmill, the coming together of the blades, hub, and rudder in the gear box converts the wind's energy into mechanical energy, resulting in the critical up and down movement of the windmill's shaft that is responsible for pumping water out of the ground. Similarly, in our model, EPPs' worldview/values, commitment to authentic engagement, and skill in attuning and connecting behaviors coalesce into a professional and meaningful relationship between themselves and parents. This relationship is critical to

DOI: 10.4324/9780429352393-8

being perceived as an EPP and contributes to the creation of a milieu of mattering that has positive outcomes for both parents and the EPPs themselves (see Chapter 11).

There are three phases involved in relationship: (1) *Establishing the Relationship*, (2) *Developing the Relationship*, and (3) *Ending the Relationship*. In addition, to maintain the connection between themselves and parents, and as part of their professional disciplinary obligations, EPPs pay particular attention to maintaining professional boundaries and they differentiate between professional and personal relationships.

Establishing the Relationship

Evidence about the importance of establishing relationships can be obtained from many sources, both within and outside health-care settings. The phenomenon of how your perception of a situation influences your behavior in that situation was well illustrated by George Schaller in his 1964 book, *The Year of the Gorilla*. Schaller, one of the world's preeminent field biologists, studied wildlife throughout Africa, Asia, and South America, and inspired Dian Fossey (famous for her own research with the endangered gorillas of the Rwandan mountain forest) with his writings. He collected far more detailed observations of the behavior of free-living gorillas than any previous scientific observer. Schaller attributed his unprecedented success to the simple fact that he had decided not to carry a rifle. This stance forced him to be sensitive to the gorillas' subtle behavioral signals and allowed him to get close to them without making them feel threatened. Earlier, less successful observers had gone into the jungle armed with rifles because they assumed (incorrectly) that gorillas were dangerously aggressive and would make unprovoked attacks.

Schaller ended up with different results because he started out from a different perspective. He assumed that the gorillas would not be dangerous as long as he treated them with respect. So, he began without a rifle and ended up discovering that he did not need one. In contrast, the ethologists who carried rifles found that they did need them. In other words, they found exactly what they had been expecting: That gorillas were too dangerous to observe closely and that sometimes they attacked and had to be shot. But these observers had created rather than discovered this confirmation of their preconceptions. It was not the gorillas' innate aggressiveness that had prompted them to attack. Rather, the observers themselves had inadvertently provoked the gorillas to attack by their thoughtlessly intrusive behavior and bearing, which was influenced by the false security and sense of invulnerability they took from their rifles.

Similar to Schaller (1964) and his approach to the gorillas, it is the EPPs' overall perspective—their worldview—that influences how they show respect to and interact with parents so that they can achieve a strong EPP–parent relationship. Specifically, EPPs recognize the interconnectivity among and between people and are committed to engaging authentically. They believe that learning parents' life circumstances is foundational to developing a trusting relationship. Within this relationship, EPPs aim to offer help in the most meaningful ways and enhance, rather than diminish, parents' well-being. EPPs see their relationship with parents as a partnership based on a dialogue of sharing complementary knowledge rather than as a one-way monologue between an expert and the other who needs fixing. In particular, EPPs believe that parents know their child best and EPPs respect parents' right to care for and make decisions about their child's care. In this light, EPPs are committed to cooperating, negotiating, and collaborating with parents to achieve their mutual goal of providing the best possible care for the child. Competent in their doing-for skills and confident in their abilities to attune and employ connecting behaviors, EPPs empower and relate to parents in meaningful ways, all the while demonstrating a natural sincerity in their encounters and developing the rapport that characterizes EPP–parent relationships—harmonious accord based on authenticity. EPPs *connect at a human level* and are *true to who they are and authentic in the situation*, which results in relationships where parents feel *in harmony* with them.

EPPs first focus with intention on *building rapport with parents to establish the relationship*. As we have noted earlier in this book, EPPs' relationship with parents begins even before meeting them—during the preparing aspect of attuning when the EPP first hears about the child/parent's situation. At that time, EPPs reflect on what thoughts, feelings, and expectations are triggered by what they initially hear about a family. They consider how they are going to respond to these triggers. Self-awareness comes into play for EPPs. They make time to be fully present with parents and to understand their world. These actions help to set the stage for the interaction and for the relationship that will form; they are integral to establishing the relationship.

Developing the Relationship

From the time of preparing for their first encounter with parents, EPPs purposefully start to build relationship. They believe that the most important thing to do during the first meeting is to show parents that they really do care, that they are committed to and are going to look after the family. They may not give verbal messages, but they *really try to make that connection because if you go in there flippantly or on the fly, it can really damage a relationship.* EPPs recognize that though this first meeting is perhaps the most devastating time for parents, it also provides a huge bonding opportunity that must not be wasted.

In addition, given the long-term nature of some of these children's conditions, EPPs recognize that the relationship they establish at the beginning is crucial because it will sustain them for months or years. Thus, from their first encounter with parents EPPs strive to create rapport with parents as an initial step toward developing a positive relationship with them. EPPs begin by greeting the parent (and child) by name and introducing themselves. They reassure parents that they *are there for them*. They pull up a chair and invite parents to tell them what is happening with the family that day. From the way they pause and lean forward expectantly, EPPs are saying, *I am ready to listen*. EPPs convey caring and commitment as an aid to later establishing trust and better relationships. They understand that if they are not sensitive in the first encounter, then parents may feel that the EPP does not care, which then threatens parents' well-being.

EPPs do care and they make this caring apparent through their posture and gestures, with their eyes and hands, when they pay close attention as parents tell their story, and in how much they nod their head in empathy. Their smile conveys understanding and encouragement just as potently as words and tells the parent that *I see you. I hear you. I'm with you*. EPPs take the time to understand parents as people and to notice subtle cues about parents' state of being. They are concerned enough to explore and understand parents' worlds because they believe that knowing about a parent is quite different from knowing the parent. Thus, EPPs are comfortable getting to know parents by engaging in polite social conversation or small talk. Parents may not always notice politeness, but they do notice rude or inconsiderate behavior, especially when their child is in a crisis situation. Small talk helps to find the common thread between EPPs and parents that fosters rapport. Parents not only expect and rely on PHCPs to care <u>for</u> their child, but they expect PHCPs to also care <u>about</u> their child and the whole family. Thus, sensing respect and authenticity in EPPs, parents invite them into the vulnerable place where their hopes and fears reside even though they know little about the EPP. In this way, the seeds of relationship are sown.

Over time, and with repeated interactions between EPPs and parents, a meaningful EPP–parent relationship evolves as all the facets of the process of attuning come together: Preparing and orienting, as well as discerning, shaping, and carrying out appropriate responses, tasks, and interventions. EPPs realize that every encounter, whether while standing in line at the coffee bar, carrying out a procedure, sharing information, or having a heart-to-heart conversation contributes to strengthening their relationship with parents. At the same time, parents continually assess EPPs' competence, sincerity, and warmth. By consistently checking with parents, EPPs reaffirm the growing trust between themselves and the parent. And through reflection, EPPs constantly assess the progress of the relationship, knowing that their behavior and awareness of their own needs, including their unconscious needs, affect the development of relationship.

Developing relationship is closely tied to parents feeling safe, having confidence in EPPs, and feeling that they are being treated with respect. Parents perceive that how EPPs build the relationship is *a combination of how quickly they've learned who we are as people, who our child is, and how to deal with us*. Parents appreciate EPPs who take the time to talk to them and their child. Parents view taking time as critical to how EPPs build connection; they compare the process to learning how to trust anyone: *If you learn how to talk to that person or make them understand what you're talking about, you throw a little bit more trust their way and they give you a little bit of respect.* In health-care settings, who EPPs are as people, how they deal with the parents, and how quickly they learn who the parents and child are as people all contribute to building a meaningful relationship.

Respect, inherent in an EPP's ability to see and treat each parent as a human being, is the basis for the trust and understanding that gets parents through the tough challenges of having a seriously ill child. In fact, lack of respect can result in more difficulties than a lack of common language. EPPs demonstrate respect through every encounter, for example, by their tone of voice, in how they address parents, and by paying attention to cultural issues. Immersed in uncertainty about what will happen, it is hard for parents to know what to do. Often feeling fearful and anxious, parents put their trust in EPPs:

> I don't even know if building good relationships is really what we did. I think it's the way that Dr. Green and nurse Julie are and how they've dealt with us. I think that's huge because we're just sitting there like deer in a set of headlights with our eyes open, waiting for them to tell us what we have to do and how we have to do it. Basically, our life is in their hands right now—they're telling us when, where, how long, and what's going to happen.

Parents' trust in EPPs leads to partnerships in the child's treatment and care and strengthens the EPP–parent relationship. EPPs understand that, ultimately, parents are the decision-makers for their child or the treatment and so they have to keep parents up to date. They affirm to parents up front that they will not hide things from them and that the parents are the voice for their child. EPPs' rapport with the children also facilitates the development of relationship with parents:

> I really respect that nurse Mena cares about my child. That's probably the thing that I like the most about her. I know she cuddles my child if I'm not there and I know that when I'm not there, she's paying attention. She's kind and reassuring to the children. If a child throws up or something like that, she's patient and it helps that she has a sense of humor.

Though EPPs develop relationship according to their individual style, once again self-awareness and self-understanding are influential in how EPPs combine their own way of being in the world with their professional encounters. The more aware EPPs are of their own personal beliefs and values, and the greater their commitment to authentic engagement, the more likely it is that there will be congruence between their intention to develop rapport and their actions to do just that.

EPPs also recognize that developing rapport is sometimes challenging, that it can be much easier to build rapport with someone who is similar to them because they can talk about a lot of things. When EPPs have little in common with parents, they recognize that working together may be harder and communication may be more difficult—but they still find it is possible. EPPs know *when parents are not gelling* with them. Nevertheless, they try to stay positive and even introduce some humor into what could be a difficult situation. Relationships with parents in such instances may not be as close as they might have been otherwise, but EPPs realize that relationships are not the same with every parent because relationships are unique, just as people are. As professionals, however, EPPs clearly develop therapeutic relationships with parents, that is, they focus on the parents' needs, not their own. Thus, each EPP's approach is individualized and strategic. They understand that good therapeutic relationships do not just happen; they need to work on them. EPPs talk about the importance of definite intent, of being aware of what they are doing and why, which is key to exemplary interaction:

> I did not tell them everything at once, but I told them enough to formulate our bond a little bit, to strengthen that bond a little bit more. You just have to decide what you're going to disclose, when you're going to disclose it, and what your intent is—what your goal is in disclosing whatever you're going to disclose. Most of the time, people just don't even think about it. Well, I'm saying think about it. Just be aware.

We found that the EPP–parent relationship also has a special quality, a special interpersonal connection that both EPPs and parents describe as a bond. Parents characterize these EPPs as authentic, warm, welcoming, real, and caring. They note that EPPs are sincere people who really listen to ensure they are on the same wavelength as parents. The special connection that EPPs have in their relationship with parents is extraordinary because of their ability to connect with and create meaningful relationships with nearly all parents.

Ending the Relationship

In addition to the strong EPP–parent relationships we encountered, we also found that EPPs recognize the time-limited or time-bound nature of professional relationships and realize that these relationships must conclude. EPPs also are aware that they need to be careful in realizing what their role is and where that role needs to end. However, not all PHCPs may understand that reality and some may not yet have learned how to end a relationship, which could contribute to them crossing professional boundaries. In their educational programs, PHCPs typically spend significant time on learning how to start relationships with a family but learning about the termination of a relationship happens less often. Yet, understanding where a relationship ends and how to make it happen makes a difference. Some EPPs talk about attending a funeral as an example of ending a relationship. They acknowledge that participating in the funeral for a baby or child they had cared for can bring closure to the relationship. At the same time, they appreciate that not everyone needs to attend the funeral as part of the termination process. They believe that each person needs to make their own decision.

EPPs, as we now discuss in this chapter, are very cognizant of needing to maintain boundaries even while recognizing the challenges they sometimes face in doing so.

Professional Relationship versus Friendship

Although EPPs are amiable and sociable, and have meaningful relationships with parents, EPPs' aim is to nurture their professional relationship, not to develop friendship with parents. While demonstrating their personal qualities and their humanity, EPPs focus on getting to know and attending to parents' needs, not their own needs. EPPs are professional in their interactions with parents: *My professional role here is to relate as a human being but not as a friend. I also think that families and patients don't actually really need or want me to be their friend.* They define their professional role as being objective about the situation in front of them while still being able to empathize with the family. At the same time, EPPs are very clear about basing their clinical practice on their own professional guidelines. They are friendly and develop good relationships, but EPPs still are able to step back and do or say what they need to.

EPPs clearly differentiate therapeutic relationships from friendships by noting that relationships with parents are formed under the very specific circumstance of a child being ill and PHCPs are present only because of their particular skills and knowledge that parents need: *You're not a friend coming in and talking about recipes with the mom—you're different from a friend because you have to be.* EPPs also recognize that parents likely come to the relationship from a more vulnerable and less powerful position than PHCPs, so EPPs see their professional focus as not only creating but also maintaining a relationship in which parents feel safe. A creative way to illustrate the difference between creating a relationship versus a friendship is to consider that *when you see a book at a bedside and say, 'Are you enjoying the book? I've read that one too', it doesn't mean you're going to invite them to your book club.* At the same time, EPPs are mindful of the challenge inherent in caring for these children and their parents. They recognize that because *we deal with really intimate subjects then sometimes, we feel really, really close to families.* Importantly, EPPs perceive maintaining boundaries as an integral aspect of their professional responsibility.

Maintaining Boundaries

The EPP–parent relationship is one where the EPP must create an environment of trust in which parents feel safe in the hands of the professional caregivers. Thus, EPPs believe that maintaining boundaries is essential because, as professionals, they must have boundaries to help the family heal or move forward. EPPs understand that they have to convey the message that they *are there for the family*. They realize that they must have an honest relationship with parents so that parents can trust their child's caregivers as professionals and to always be professional. Separating professional and personal boundaries does not mean though that EPPs are impersonal or distant in relating to parents. EPPs are friendly, engaging, and take an interest in parents' lives while still remaining professional. However, they view something like attending a family's house for dinner as going down a slippery slope. They believe they need to be cautious and not start on that slope. Most parents too do not want to cross the boundary nor do they want PHCPs to cross it. They believe that maintaining boundaries is about confidentiality and respect for them and their family.

It sometimes happens that the lives of parents and PHCPs will overlap outside of the hospital. EPPs give careful thought to how to handle such situations, for example:

> I have cared for babies whose parents are parents at my kid's school and I realized, 'I cannot be talking with that parent about what happens in the unit.' I can talk about parent things when I am with them in a parent situation, I can ask how their child is doing, as any parent might, but I cannot talk with them about things that happened in the unit with their child or anyone else's child. We need to be very clear in our minds about our role on the unit and then our role if we see that person outside of the unit.

It is clear that while retaining their professionalism, EPPs manage to put their heart as well as their mind into their relationship with parents. In fact, it is this combination of heart and mind that helps to sustain the therapeutic relationship and the bond EPPs have with parents. At the same time, EPPs also recognize that it is normal to be affected and saddened by what happens, particularly when children die. But EPPs learn to incorporate this reality into the way they view their work. They acknowledge that it gets emotional, but they learn to create their own boundaries because they know they have to if they want to be able to continue in this field without becoming burnt out. EPPs have come to realize that *it is not their dance, it is the parents' dance, and it is their job to guide the parents, not to be them.* They understand that if they stop being affected by this work, if they do not feel sad or angry or upset with the stories they hear and the things they see, they should not do this work. So, they do not define boundaries as what they are feeling. Rather, they know that they need to deal with the immediate situation while being aware of their feelings and then later reflect on the experience and sit with their feelings.

EPPs are successful at maintaining boundaries because they are able to differentiate the personal from the professional aspects of their lives by using an internal monitor developed through self-awareness, rather than relying solely on external rules. This internal aspect comes from reflecting on and learning from their experience; it involves maturational learning. Some EPPs note that, based on their own experience, dealing with the challenges of maintaining boundaries may be more difficult for younger and less experienced PHCPs: *I think that every clinician here will tell you that they had one kid who broke their heart, and that child teaches you to be better at setting your boundaries.* But as we have noted in Chapter 7 of this book, age is not a defining characteristic of exemplary practice; such practice has more to do with the level of maturity that comes from reflecting on and learning from your experiences. External rules in the form of policies and guidelines are helpful for students and new PHCPs, for more experienced PHCPs who are still clarifying their personal codes of conduct, and at times for EPPs. However, EPPs are guided by their internal rules. They understand that there is a difference between *I cannot come to your house for dinner because the rules say I cannot do that* versus *I cannot come to your house for dinner because I personally do not do that.* In the first situation, the person is guided by something external (which does not imply that falling back on rules is necessarily a problem); in the second, the person is guided by something internal—learning about boundaries has been internalized. Having clear rules of personal conduct facilitates EPPs separating their personal from their professional responsibilities and enables them to keep clear boundaries without compromising caring and compassion.

EPPs take seriously their professional responsibility to adhere to the standards for maintaining boundaries that are set by their professional associations and colleges and that warn against personal involvement compromising therapeutic relationships. Though EPPs find these guidelines worthwhile, they do not rely on them as replacements for their own moral compass for doing what is right. They understand that boundaries should not always be rule-governed; boundary negotiation requires professional judgment. Characteristic of EPPs is their commitment to their own ethical and moral integrity, to their own personal codes of conduct, and to how they face the challenges of maintaining boundaries.

Challenges to Maintaining Boundaries

Maintaining boundaries is not always easy, especially because the development of a strong relationship implies getting to know specific details about the parent. EPPs find that several challenges present themselves, and they must rely on their own internal rules of personal conduct that define their boundaries.

Cultural Expectations

Health-care settings are diverse and PHCPs encounter families from a variety of backgrounds in their daily work. Sometimes, parents can be very insistent in their desire to show gratitude for the care they have received, for example, by inviting a doctor or nurse to dinner in their home. EPPs recognize that they need to gracefully discourage such insistence while also acknowledging and accepting that there are sometimes cultural differences that account for some parents' wishes. However, EPPs understand that complying would be unwise professionally. Moreover, EPPs recognize that parents need a PHCP who is going to be their doctor, their nurse, and so on, not their friend. Thus, EPPs are friendly and engage with parents while still retaining professional boundaries.

PHCPs' Personal Circumstances

Personal circumstances, such as caring for a parent with dementia, living alone as a newcomer to this country, or having children of their own may influence how PHCPs' boundaries are maintained. It is especially hard for some PHCPs who have a child the same age as the sick child, but other PHCPs find that after having a family of their own, it is easier to differentiate work from home and establish a good balance between them.

Long-Term Relationships With Families

Caring for families over long periods of time also can present a special kind of challenge: For example, it can be hard for PHCPs to draw the line between what is appropriate versus inappropriate when caring for the same baby every shift for months on end. The boundaries can become complicated and confusing because the PHCP becomes very close with these families. However, EPPs recognize that although it is definitely a challenge, they still maintain boundaries.

Working with children who have complex, chronic conditions means that EPPs are often with these families when the child is dying, and they are intimately involved with the parents. But, even during the dying process and then afterward, the connection does not lead to friendships for EPPs: *The mother doesn't need my clinical services anymore, but she often stops by to say hello and we have chitchat moments. But there wouldn't be a clinical reason why I would get engaged.* Experience with getting close to a child or parents results in EPPs learning how to deal with this type of situation: They recognize their hurt when the child dies and they realize that trying to block that sadness may lead to building a wall that impairs their ability to relate optimally to other children and their families in the future. So EPPs consciously do not block their sadness; they recognize their own limits and take action to ensure time for personal recovery, for example, by listening to their body, being aware of their responses, and if they feel they have reached their limit for right now, by stepping away from the situation.

Gift-Giving

Gift-giving presents another challenge for boundaries because of the implications inherent in the act and the potential impact on the relationship between PHCPs and parents. EPPs noted that gift-giving holds the potential of significantly affecting the PHCP–parent relationship and may lead to the PHCP showing or being perceived to show favoritism or feeling obligated to those parents who provide gifts. EPPs realize that some parents just want to show their appreciation, but EPPs think that it is better to reject personal gifts. Some parents may have a different perspective:

> I don't see anything wrong with giving gifts. You could look at it as if they're just doing their job—yeah, they are, but in all honesty, a taxi driver does his job and you give him a tip and he's not doing anything special, he's just driving from point A to B. Here, it's your kid's welfare, so these people who are really helping you out or are helping you cope, I see no problem bringing them coffees and cookies, and stuff like that—why not? I think having a good rapport with these people is a good thing.

This parent's argument makes sense for small gifts meant for the staff, but she also expressed another motive:

> Obviously, even if you don't have a good relationship with them, they're taking care of the kids. It's like that old saying that you catch more bees with honey than you do with vinegar. I'm not saying you're trying to bribe them but being nice or having some sort of connection with these people—if anything brings you closer, the care, I believe, is even better.

Some EPPs support a strict no-gifts policy that would help PHCPs know how to handle gift-giving situations, but they also allow that such a rule might not be understood or could be insulting to some parents, particularly those from a culture in which gift-giving is a common way of saying thank you. EPPs do not want to offend parents, so sometimes they say that PHCPs are not allowed to accept gifts and could be seriously reprimanded for doing so. Other approaches include suggesting to the parent that if they want to do something to help the program, then they could donate to a related charity. The nature of the gift and to whom it would go also play a role in whether or not EPPs accept a gift—for example, chocolates would be something that the whole team could share, whereas money could be put toward something like a baby clothing fund as a thank you from the family, so the whole unit would benefit. Other EPPs recognize that accepting a parent's gift can be beneficial because it can strengthen the friendly relationship between themselves and a parent, add to a parent's self-worth, and prevent the parent from feeling hurt or offended if the gift were to be rejected. EPPs agree that if they had a policy that was clear to both PHCPs <u>and</u> families, then challenges with gift-giving might be avoided or alleviated.

Social Media

Social media is a significant challenge for PHCPs in maintaining boundaries. The use of email, becoming friends on Facebook, and other evolving ways that people communicate electronically is a rapidly changing landscape and one in which increasing numbers of people are participating. Today's ability to have instant communication and to have very little privacy raise issues for EPPs. For example, they now have to deal with PHCPs or other colleagues communicating by Facebook and accidentally or deliberately including information about patients in their posts: *Now, we most definitely have to stop people from even thinking about including material about patients.* Unfortunately, communication has become so instant that people are talking about whatever they are currently doing: '*I'm going to the grocery store. I'm going to run an IV for baby.*' *Oops! It's crossed the boundary.* Twitter is a hot issue. PHCPs and volunteers on Facebook sometimes friend themselves with one of their patients. Boundary and confidentiality issues are on the rise.

EPPs' challenges with social media may arise because of some parents, and especially teenagers, who view this way of communicating as normal and natural and who may become confused or even bewildered when another person (including PHCPs) will not participate. Some EPPs simply deal with social media by having nothing to do with it. In some situations, they resort to a policy issue, citing that the hospital does not allow the use of social media or that their professional regulating body (e.g., the College of Nurses) does not condone the use of it. Though initially some EPPs were reluctant to decline invites because they were worried about hurting someone's feelings, they now realize that they must decline to protect their own professionalism.

Many technological safeguards are already in place within the health-care system, so perhaps part of the challenge is to develop ways and means to effectively use existing safeguards to monitor and manage communication flow. Policies regarding social media have had to be implemented at times to protect the safety, privacy, and confidentiality of patients, but to a certain extent, some decisions will probably remain personal and each individual will have to act according to their personal beliefs and wishes. For the most part, social media is unregulated, and it is always up to individuals to use it in ways that they deem appropriate. Privacy settings, for example, are always a matter of personal choice, and EPPs are careful about their own boundaries.

EPPs constantly guard against infractions, for example, the posting of pictures of families or children on their personal pages, but they also educate families who may not understand these things. To complicate social media matters further, there are levels of engagement and nuances that need to be explained and adhered to. For example, providing a patient or parent with a personal email address may be off limits, whereas offering a professional hospital-based email may be totally acceptable. It may not be appropriate to give a private cell phone number to a family, but a hospital-based number used to contact that EPP/PHCP may be freely given out. Too deep a level of engagement with families via social media may result in relationships based on favoritism, which is problematic:

> Any time as a professional we start choosing families that become special to us, which is one result of what happens when social media is used in a personal way, is problematic. I always remind staff who are having these issues that the family who might not speak English very well, the family who may not be the most well-liked family, what does that mean for them? Do they receive what they need? Are you available in the same way to the families that may be 'difficult'?

Guidelines are in place about the use of social media, but even when used and followed, they may not suffice. EPPs agree that if there is a problem with crossing boundaries of any sort, it is up to them, and not families, to clarify things and to make sure that the relationship remains appropriately professional, *Sometimes I wish there were more rigid guidelines, but then at the same time we're grown professionals, we should know, right?*

Other Strategies for Maintaining Boundaries

For EPPs, the significant risk of crossing boundaries with parents means that they would then be treating those parents differently from others. Given EPPs' broad perspective on humankind and their valuing of social justice, they see differential treatment as less than optimal care and as compromising their own integrity. EPPs also warn against the negative effects on PHCPs themselves of not maintaining boundaries because, over time, those PHCPs may find themselves in emotional turmoil or difficult circumstances; eventually, they may experience burnout. To avoid these potential risks, EPPs offered some clear but simple strategies for maintaining boundaries.

EPPs remember that they *would never have met this family without coming together as a practitioner with the child and family*. This focus helps them maintain their role as a PHCP and the parent retains their role, which means each can share things appropriately. For EPPs, relationships with parents start and end in the hospital, and contact outside of the hospital (family home, restaurant, coffee shop, etc.) is out of bounds. The hospital or work setting provides a clear, natural, and geographic boundary for maintaining professional relationships. EPPs are particularly aware that the work they do in accompanying families can be not just exhausting; it also can really break their heart. But it is precisely because the work is so difficult that they know they must be aware of how staying in the mode of PHCP may be challenging. They understand that, because they are human beings, the personal and the professional mesh to some extent. Adhering to geographical spaces aids in not taking their work home with them, allowing EPPs to draw clear boundaries between their work and homelife. As we mentioned in Chapter 7, intentionally creating transition time while traveling between work and home is an effective way of differentiating their personal and professional lives.

EPPs excel at gently but firmly setting geographic boundaries with parents. For example, some families still visit EPPs in the hospital after their child died years ago, but only after they have first received the EPP's permission. These visits are restricted, for example, to once a year or so, and if parents bring treats, then they know they need to be for all the staff. EPPs who decline an invitation for coffee might instead invite the parent to update them on how they or their baby is doing. They let the parent know that they are welcome to use the EPP's work email, but they do not share their personal email. If an EPP receives a card to their work email, for example, about a baby's first year or a big milestone, they simply will write back saying, *It's so great to see you guys are doing well, my best wishes.* But that is all they do.

Maintaining boundaries does not preclude EPPs recognizing the potential value of continuing connection with parents—but within the bounds of the physical space and for a specific reason that is therapeutic for the family. For example, PHCPs welcome parents of neonates who return to the NICU to proudly and gratefully show off their now-thriving baby, and hospice staff interact with families, including bereaved parents, at regular gatherings that celebrate families and staff, for example, the annual Christmas tree-lighting ceremony or garden teas. However, even those boundaries occasionally need flexibility. For example, sometimes parents will invite staff to participate in a family celebration, such as a neonate reaching her first birthday or a terminally ill child becoming an adolescent on his 13th birthday. Being in contact with parents outside of the setting is perceived as acceptable if done as part of a group, so being open and not secretive about it, but not if done individually. Such events do not necessarily lead to ongoing communications with the parents; often it is a one-time contact only.

Another strategy for maintaining boundaries is that EPPs seek support in maintaining their professional perspective by remembering they are part of a team. Because the team has the responsibility of caring for all of the parents, then it is not the responsibility of individual EPPs to take on alone the challenges of any individual parent's situation. So when they are at work, they are there 100%. They realize that they are not the only person who works there and that the care is given by all of the team. The workplace environment also is a major source of support for maintaining balance. EPPs believe that establishing a work-based social support network to debrief, share, and talk about what is going on is invaluable in helping them continue their work. EPPs also recommend having normal relationships, a support system outside of work, because that too is a beneficial strategy for maintaining boundaries.

Finally, self-awareness is the foundational strategy for maintaining boundaries. EPPs are committed to establishing meaningful relationships with parents and they invest heavily in doing so professionally. But they also admit to being affected personally by the emotional nature of their work: *If you carry every single emotional situation, you can't do this line of work.* EPPs believe that crossing boundaries is most often the result of PHCPs meeting their own needs and not those of the parents. Thus, clarifying whose need is being met underlies EPPs' basic strategy of frequently checking in with themselves to ensure they know whether it is their need or the parent's need that guides their work. EPPs suggest that figuring out the balance between their professional and personal life is an ongoing reflective process:

> I aim to not lose myself in the work and that's partly about self-awareness and partly about my own integrity. I've had to work at learning that and at developing awareness and growth. But I think it's definitely part of my work—understanding where I begin and end, and where the other begins and ends, and yet being able to create a connection that's meaningful within us being two separate entities. The connection we create is very meaningful and very important.

Further Thoughts on Relationships and Boundaries

Inherent in EPPs' worldview and values is the idea that persons have a basic human dignity deserving of respect. Respect is at the heart of the EPP–parent relationship. Respect can be interpreted as approaching another person (or a group, idea, or an object) with regard or esteem. It says, you matter and I care about you, messages that EPPs convey to parents through their words and their behavior as they *establish relationships* and create rapport. Consider the relevant questions in Box 8.1 as you think about how you develop rapport and build strong relationships. Remember too that rapport is all about finding similarities and being on the same wavelength as somebody else. Being empathic can help you achieve rapport, as can reflecting back to parents what you have heard them say and clarifying what people say to you. However, quite a lot of rapport-building happens without words and through nonverbal communication channels. If there is a mismatch between what you are saying and your body language, parents will believe the body language. Consider how you develop rapport with people who are different from you. When you have the opportunity to meet with people who are different from yourself, reflect on the interaction and identify what went well, or not, so that you can apply your learning in subsequent encounters.

Self-awareness plays a critical role in developing rapport, establishing strong relationships, and maintaining boundaries. Therefore, it is important

Box 8.1: Relationships and Boundaries: Questions for Consideration

Relationships

- Do I use safe topics for initial small talk, such as the weather, or perhaps how parents traveled to the hospital?
- Do I listen to what parents are saying and look for shared experiences or circumstances?
- How do I show that I can see the parent's point of view?
- Can I find something to laugh about together with the parents?
- Am I conscious of my body positioning, body movements, eye contact, facial expressions, and tone of voice as I build rapport with another person?
- How do I develop rapport with people who are different from me as I navigate an increasingly diverse and complex world?
- Am I aware of the personal circumstances or encounters that may be influencing how I am able to develop strong relationships and maintain boundaries?
- How do I maintain the difference between my professional role versus a friendship?
- How do I deal with the closeness that sometimes develops for me with children and parents?
- What have I learned about ending relationships with patients and parents?
- How do I typically end a professional relationship with families?

Boundaries

- Have I ever crossed any boundaries in ongoing relationships with families? If so, what happened?
- How do I maintain my boundaries?
- What specific behaviors do I engage in for the purpose of separating my professional and personal lives?
- How do I decide what I am going to disclose to parents about myself? What is my goal in choosing what to disclose?
- What do I think about using my work setting as a geographic boundary for maintaining professional relationships?
- How do I use my team to help in maintaining boundaries?
- How aware am I of professional organizations' and work settings' guidelines about boundaries, social media, and gift giving? Do I find them helpful?

Social Media

- What strategies do I use to ensure privacy for myself and others?
- How do I handle issues of confidentiality?
- What are the safeguards in my setting that I can use to monitor and manage the flow of communication?

Gift-Giving

- When thinking about a time I was offered a gift, did I sense that the gift was given to secure preferential treatment?
- Whether I declined or accepted the gift, what were the reasons for my choice? How was my relationship with the parent altered by my response?
- Do I have a personal rule for accepting gifts—never, always, or sometimes depending on the circumstance? How has my rule worked for me?
- What kind of circumstances lead to me refusing a gift?

that you make the time to think not only about what you are doing but also why you are doing it. Many EPPs say that their experiences of caring for seriously ill and dying children has changed them in significant ways. Has that been the case for you? If so, what happened? People's actions and thoughts also derive from how they perceive the work they do. EPPs are committed to their work as a career and believe that they are contributing to a greater goal or mission. Do you see your work as a long-term career? Or as a temporary job? Do you find joy in your work? Do you see yourself as part of a team?

Caring for the same patients and families over time can sometimes blur the lines of these relationships. Consider how you separate your professional role from a friendship and how you deal with closeness between you and families. It can be particularly difficult to *end a relationship* with patients and parents who have had prolonged stays in the hospital. Have you ever maintained a friendship with a parent past the time of the child's discharge? If so, what happened?

Crossing professional boundaries may be an undesirable result of getting too close to a family. EPPs have several strategies for maintaining their boundaries, for example, using mutual sharing to establish a good connection but being choosey about what they share. Think about the boundary questions in Box 8.1 as you consider behaviors you engage in to separate your professional and personal lives. Online communications can help establish positive relationships but can also make it easier to cross boundaries.

Think about how you use social media with children, parents, and colleagues and how you maintain privacy and confidentiality while managing the flow of communication.

Appreciative parents may present their PHCPs with gifts, an apparently simple act that can raise complex issues in the care relationship and may be a time when boundaries are crossed. Professional organizations and work settings typically have guidelines regarding boundaries, using social media, or gift-giving. How aware are you of these guidelines, and do you find them helpful?

The ethical core of each health-care discipline is the therapeutic relationship between the practitioner and the patient. Indeed, our study has shown this to be true as illustrated by our windmill. It is the motion of the shaft in a windmill that draws the water, whereas it is the relationship between parents and PHCPs that draws out the milieu of mattering that contributes to outcomes for practitioners and parents alike. Moreover, just as all parts of the windmill are necessary for the movement of the shaft, so too are all parts of our model necessary for the relationship. But there is still more to the story, namely the parts that are outside of the windmill itself. We discuss those contextual influencing factors in the next two chapters.

References

Council of Accountable Physician Practices. (2017). *2017 consumer health care priorities study: What patients and doctors want from the health care system. Focus group research results.* http://accountablecaredoctors.org/wp-content/uploads/2017/11/capp-research_what-patients-and-doctors-want.pdf

Frank, A. (2004). *The renewal of generosity: Illness, medicine and how to live.* University of Chicago Press.

Schaller, G. B. (1964). *The year of the gorilla.* University of Chicago Press.

9 Setting and Teamwork Contextual Factors

A real team, a team that functions best, means that the difficult questions, the things people are thinking, are said aloud. It's creating the feeling that everyone is heard and not in a placating way. People can speak openly, talk about things, and move to a place of coming to a common agreement on a situation or an approach. Another characteristic is treating yourselves with respect. Respect is foundational to listening to one another. Team members aren't judged for expressing their own view, don't have to fear saying, 'I don't understand this,' or 'I don't agree with that,' or 'What about this?' If you can do that, it creates something where people begin to understand another perspective that's outside of their own and it's all on the table and everyone is focused on the child and family. It isn't just the plan of care, it's a common place of understanding, especially in ethical decisions that come up. I do believe that a good strong team is centered around the best for the child and family and does not operate in silos.

In our attempt to understand exemplary interaction, we realized it was not enough to only describe the actions of EPPs and the role of personal factors for EPPs. We must also ask: In what surroundings does the EPP practice? The impact of the environment or context is critical—the social environment has this power because people do not exist apart from a society. EPPs, like all PHCPs who work in health-care settings, do not work in isolation. As we show in our model, EPPs are likely to be affected by what is going on beyond them as individual clinicians—the setting in which they work, the health-care team of which they are a part, the health-care institution where they are situated, and the particular societal factors within which they are located—just as a windmill is also affected by the environment. To operate optimally, a windmill must be located on stable terrain. But even when fixed on sturdy ground, a prairie windmill is subjected to nature's whims of rain, snow, ice, and heat—the climactic conditions that continuously surround and impact the windmill and the ground on which it sits. Fortunately, windmills are well-constructed to withstand such factors.

EPPs are by our definition solidly grounded in their practice, but they too must be able to withstand the surrounding factors that can negatively affect their ability to practice in the way they want to. On the other hand, those same factors—the setting/team within which they work, their institutional

DOI: 10.4324/9780429352393-9

context, including the leadership within the institution and setting, and their broader society—also can contribute to facilitating EPPs' exemplary practice. In this chapter and the next, we will discuss how these surrounding factors can both constrain and enhance the practice of PHCPs. Our specific focus in this chapter is on the group of factors that is particular to the immediate work environment, that is, *Settings* and *Teamwork*.

Settings in Our Study

The inclusion in our project of three separate pediatric settings (NICU, oncology, and hospice) provided an unusual opportunity to observe and analyze different organizational team structures, communication patterns, and approaches to care, all of which we discovered arose from the overall priority for care in each setting. Examining the settings themselves allowed us to not only understand that EPPs value their interactions within their teams but also identify how EPPs contribute significantly to their team's optimal functioning. Most importantly, we also were able to see that EPPs could be identified regardless of the differences in the settings where they worked or in the teams to which they belonged. EPPs shared this underlying similarity even though the physical environment of each setting and institution differed considerably. EPPs and parents alike recognized the challenges of their particular setting but tended not to focus on them. Rather, in NICU and oncology they adapted to crowded and sometimes noisy conditions as best they could and eagerly anticipated the new hospital under construction that would house a new NICU and oncology unit. In the hospice, EPPs sometimes struggled with problems such as slanted floors due to the age of the building, but they also appreciated the open spaces that were uncrowded, quiet, and peaceful, particularly when a child was dying.

To help you understand—and perhaps identify with—our settings, we briefly describe these settings and their team structures, with the caveat that we are not claiming any one type of team as better or worse than another; they are simply different from one another and there is no right team. In general, an important difference between the settings was in the priority for care in each setting, which in turn affected the team structure.

NICU

Since the early 1960s, progressively enhanced technology has made the viability of newborns possible at an increasingly earlier gestational age. These fragile little ones are the target of care in NICU where the priority is to save the neonates' lives. The instability and rapidly changing condition of these infants often requires urgent decision-making about high-level, technical interventions carried out at the side of specialized incubators or cribs located within the NICU. As babies of progressively younger gestational age can now be saved, the number of babies needing care has increased dramatically. Thus, the NICU setting at the time of the study is very large, comprising 60 beds within an open space so that all babies can be under watchful eyes simultaneously. Timing is critical, the pace is rapid, and the atmosphere can be tense. PHCPs focus on the numerous tasks related to the babies' physical care. The team structure comprises a cluster of sub-teams, all of which are part of a larger group to which every discipline offers input as needed to save the newborn's life. Thus, the team is symbolized by numerous circles, each representing a different discipline, that overlap to varying degrees (see Figure 9.1).

Nursing is divided into 10 teams. Within each nursing team, nurses cover for one another to provide continuous care to their patients, partially using a primary nursing model.[1] Respiratory therapists (RT), occupational therapists, social workers, and medical consultants are called in as needed for any particular child. Attending physicians rotate on a predetermined two-week on-call schedule and, during their rotation, provide medical care to groups of children; they are not identified as the primary physician for any children. The arrows on Figure 9.1 indicate that communication goes back and forth between and among circles (e.g., nursing and RT, or medicine and nursing) but not necessarily to the entire group. Of course, the size of teams tends to make a difference in team dynamics. A small team working together daily often has more opportunities to develop trust and understanding than does a larger group of rotating individuals.

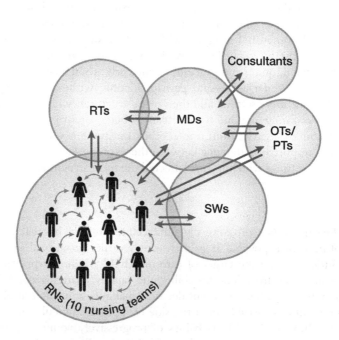

Figure 9.1 Neonatal Intensive Care Team Structure

Oncology

Advances in the field of oncology (e.g., chemotherapy and radiation) have made cure possible for many children with cancer. Treatment is aimed at cure and typically follows standardized, controlled protocols administered during brief hospital stays. Care is targeted to the child and parents. PHCPs' ultimate goal is to get families home safely so that after treatment they live healthy, happy lives. Although there are critical times during the course of treating a child's cancer, the pace in oncology settings is relatively slower than in the NICU and the environment is less tense. The oncology setting comprises 24 beds, divided into two units on separate floors with one above the other and joined by stairways and elevators. Patients are in separate rooms; at least one parent is required to stay with a child as much as possible. Upon admission, a child is seen by an oncologist and nurse clinician who, along with a social worker, remain as that child's primary team for the duration of the child's care, which can extend over months to years. Thus, the oncology team (see Figure 9.2) is represented by concentric circles, with the primary oncologist, nurse clinician, and social worker as the inner circle or core of the team. The next circle includes bedside nurses, child life specialists, and pharmacists. In the outermost circle are allied health workers (e.g., physio- and occupational therapists) whose expertise is sought depending on the needs of the particular child as determined by the primary team. Everyone

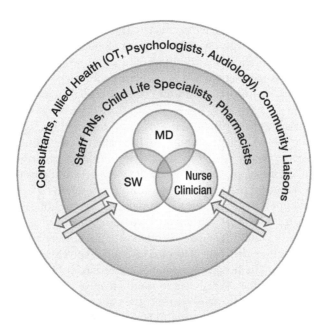

Figure 9.2 Pediatric Oncology Unit Team Structure

else (e.g., the medical colleagues of the primary physician, medical residents and students, consultants, or community physicians) is also in this outer circle. Communication flows freely back and forth within the center circle, with input from the outer circle when required by the primary team.

Hospice

Despite the advances that enable many newborns and children to survive, not all children with CCCs can be cured. The goal of hospice care is to support these children and their families during disease progression through to peaceful death and then bereavement. PHCPs value being with families when they are at their most vulnerable and accompanying them on their journey. Treatment and responses to it are unpredictable for a wide range of conditions, requiring time for family members to figure things out for all aspects (e.g., physical, psychosocial, and spiritual) of their lives. Thus, the pace is slower than for the other two settings. Moreover, inherent in hospice care is the fostering of a relaxed, comfortable environment. The hospice, a four-story renovated mansion, has beds for eight children plus two suites for families. The hospice is located in a quiet, urban residential setting and is surrounded by a large garden and play area. Also inherent in hospice philosophy is teamwork, as demonstrated by the composition of the steering committee that developed the hospice. This committee had parent, physician, social work, child life, and academic and clinical nursing representation. As a result, the hospice team is conceptualized as all staff who have contact with the families, including staff who might not be considered part of a team elsewhere, such as the cook and housekeeper. In addition, volunteers are an important adjunct to the team. This team is represented as a pie diagram with each discipline as one piece of the pie. Communication flows back and forth across the pie (see Figure 9.3).

Given the various factors involved, it is to be expected that teams would operate differently in each setting. Additionally, each setting's historical development has played a role in determining team structure. In both oncology and neonatology, treating acute illness was the impetus for specialized medical attention that occurred at a time when the traditional medical model—based upon a physician leader with allied health professionals playing a supporting role—was the norm. Over time, teams in these settings have become more interdisciplinary as other disciplines were invited to play a more central part of the team. Hospice care is a relatively newer development in pediatrics. The hospice model is characterized by a flatter hierarchy of professional roles that contributes to more effective access to knowledge from all members on the team. Over time, the cultures of the medical model and the hospice model have become integrated (Youngwerth & Twaddle, 2011) to create more egalitarian models in which the contributions of each discipline are equally valued and recognized.

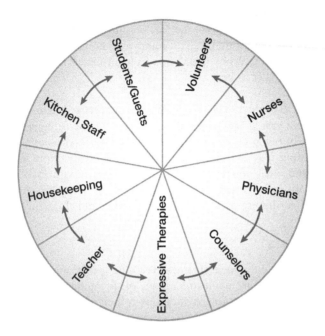

Figure 9.3 Pediatric Hospice Team Structure

Importance of Fit Between EPPs and Their Setting

Across settings, EPPs share the perception that they fit with the goal or mission of their particular setting and with the way their team works. Their personal beliefs align with the kinds of things they do in their work:

> When I first visited here and went to rounds, I thought, 'You know, this is like a gold mine—to find a team that works as a team.' To actually be together, planning together, with a variety of disciplines—I see it very rarely in health care. And so right there, that sort of was a big hook for me. I thought, 'Oh, I can fit here.'

In each place, EPPs commented on how staff must have a particular way of being in the world to work there. EPPs had found their place, sometimes after leaving other settings they had not liked. As well, EPPs mentioned that some PHCPs had left the setting when they found the work, or the nature of the team, was not a fit for them. Those PHCPs usually left with the support of leaders who recognized the lack of fit and encouraged them to not feel embarrassed or ashamed that they could not do that type of work because it is not for everybody. EPPs tend to describe working in their setting as their dream job. They love all parts of their job: Working with families, their team members, that they are still being challenged, and that there is room for them to grow; they are comfortable with where they are.

EPPs have the self-awareness to recognize when they fit and why; their heart is in their work. When members of a team share that passion for their work, teamwork is at its best:

> I think one of the biggest pieces when I first started here was the philosophy of caring for the families and care for the caregiver. Having a practice of being contemplative about your work was built-in, such as the coming together and checking in emotionally about how you're doing and what you're doing. And you practice with each other that stance of nonjudgment, of compassion, and so if we can do that with each other, then we can do that with families and children.

Pride in Teamwork

Regardless of the differences in the development of teams in each setting, EPPs are proud of their own team's unique quality and they love their team. If they are not sure about or are questioning their practice or feel that they did not do something right with the family, they know they have someone else to bounce ideas off, which they perceive as being unusual based on their previous experiences. Interestingly, EPPs in each setting view their own team and specialty area as unique and draw comparisons with other settings. They feel very lucky to be working in their own unique area.

However, perceptions of team could vary considerably—as discovered by EPPs who had occasion to work in settings other than their own where they saw differences in how physicians ruled (or not) the team, as well as how the input of various disciplines was sought and received. EPPs also acknowledge that some people are better team players than others. EPPs realize that though some PHCPs may identify themselves as members of a team, it seems to be only a matter of speaking the words rather than a conscientious awareness of teamwork:

> If a person has their area of expertise and focuses only on that without negotiating, discussing, or developing plans of care together, then simply saying, 'We are a team' or 'I am a member of this team' does not result in an optimally functioning team.

EPPs note that teamwork requires explicit attentiveness. People cannot just claim they are a team; rather, they have to focus on making a team, deciding how it works, and telling others that they are building a team and this is what it means to work here. EPPs explicitly tell new colleagues that they have joined a team. EPPs are astutely aware of the value of well-functioning teams and they purposefully focus on facilitating optimal functioning of their own team.

EPPs' Contributions to Optimal Teamwork

EPPs' worldview/values and commitment to authentic engagement provide the foundation for how they are in the world. Believing that all human beings are worthy of respect and dignity, EPPs perceive their colleagues as fellow human beings, similar to how they perceive parents, and they interact with their team members in similar ways to how they interact with parents. For example, EPPs make a concerted effort to orient by welcoming young or inexperienced staff members and students to the norms, rules, and mores of the setting. In addition, by seeking their colleagues' perspectives, EPPs get to know them as people, to understand their colleagues' strengths and limitations:

> If there's something I don't understand, I will ask, 'Okay, you're saying this, why do you want to do that?' I find that it makes for a better environment because people feel like they're listened to or appreciated and next steps can be clarified.

Thus, EPPs can more easily discern what matters most in the moment for their colleague(s). EPPs shape their responses accordingly, for example, by thoughtfully congratulating colleagues on a job well done, by willingly teaching others whose knowledge may be lacking, such as about various cultural patterns of behavior, or by mentoring others in finessing their various skills. EPPs reflect, both individually and with team members, on their interactions with one another. Undeniably, in these interactions with their colleagues EPPs enact all facets of the attuning process along with the eight connecting behaviors, just as they do with parents.

EPPs contribute much to the team's optimal functioning and are frequently seen by other team members as role models or leaders. They do not necessarily hold formal positions of leadership, but when they do they make exemplary leaders. Not all PHCPs strive to become EPPs and not all EPPs strive to assume management or administrative positions. But optimal team functioning is dependent upon managers and administrators having a conscientious awareness of team and what makes it work, as well as having exemplary interaction abilities. EPPs note that different leadership styles have different impacts. They believe that the extent to which they work well together as a team and as PHCPs depends on leadership—people's own philosophy and the leader's philosophy.

Optimal team functioning may require that the team is led not always by the same person but by the team member who is the most appropriate leader for the particular situation, and EPPs are willing to take on such roles as appropriate. EPPs also understand that teams have dual but interrelated purposes—to facilitate patient care and to support a positive working environment for the PHCPs. Regardless of their formal or informal position as leaders, EPPs intentionally facilitate the achievement of both purposes by being explicitly attentive to activities that help to create and maintain optimal team functioning.

Creating a Safe Environment

A team is where PHCPs can brainstorm and share ideas, speak up, be heard, feel respected, and count on one another; otherwise, they only have a group or a so-called team of people, but it is not functioning as a team. For EPPs, optimal team functioning is evident in how team members describe their team and teamwork to each other and to new staff and students when they tell them that they are building a team. EPPs also let parents know what team means in the setting:

> The care is a shared thing by the team. One example would be that if parents say to me, 'You're the only nurse who can look after my child,' I would know that's a huge issue because that does not benefit me or the family. So it's important to say, 'Pierre needs to be taken care of by all of the team and this is how we do it here. If you have specific concerns about somebody, then we need to know how we can address those concerns so that person can provide the best possible care to your child.' Reliance on one person is not what we do, we really encourage connections with others.

Such a strong sense of trust in their team can occur only when everyone's competence is expected and ensured, but a safe environment is also required.

A safe environment comes about not by chance, but by conscious choice and planning. EPPs strive to create such an atmosphere. To EPPs, a safe work environment is not about ladders falling down or equipment breaking; it is about workplace safety in the sense of it being safe to share their emotion as team members. A safe environment enables team members to feel comfortable in speaking out, to share their own emotions, struggles, or successes, and to engage in dialogue. Such mutual exchange creates opportunities for team members to figure things out, plan, understand various points of view, and come to a common understanding of an approach to care. Working with the same team over an extended period of time provides more opportunities to communicate with one another regularly, facilitates the formation of relationships among members, and enhances members' ability to work together. Longevity and consistency in working together foster respect and trust and allow team members to work in sync—they know what each other does and how they do it, and they can anticipate and rely upon colleagues doing what they should. EPPs value being able to approach anybody in their team. They know each other's style and what is going on. For example, if someone is working closely with a family whose child is not doing well or has died, they all gauge the situation and help one another.

EPPs advocate for and support attendance at regularly scheduled meetings as an avenue to help team members know one another and to establish trust, respect, and relationship. To achieve these outcomes, however, EPPs emphasize that the people with the needed expertise must be included in relevant team meetings. They expect a good representation of clinical people at meetings when setting team goals for the future. EPPs want parents to attend meetings when the team is trying to make changes so that what they are trying to change works with what a parent would want or need for their child. They emphasize the importance of making sure to have clinical staff on a project team when something new is going to be implemented. And if something has happened at the bedside or the team is trying to understand what is not working at the bedside, then the clinical staff should always be asked for their story about what they think would make things better, because they typically have the answer. EPPs show respect for their colleagues—a key ingredient for optimal team functioning.

Demonstrating Respect

EPPs demonstrate respect even in seemingly little ways, such as when everyone's presence is acknowledged at the start of meetings. If members, new people, and guests are introduced by their names, not solely by their roles, they are more likely to feel they belong:

> It is funny to see how such a simple gesture as introductions is so significant to me because I have been to many meetings where this is not done. It sends the message that everyone in the team knows who everyone is and what their role is.

Respect is also shown when members' opinions are acknowledged and appreciated. EPPs know that people feel part of the team when others appreciate their experience, for example, when a PHCP says something about what they think and their colleagues hear it. And vice versa when someone asks a colleague what they think about an issue. EPPs recognize that when someone feels their opinion is valued, they feel on equal footing with their colleagues.

Additionally, EPPs show respect by seeking to learn about what is involved in their colleagues' roles. They then use that information to help themselves become a better nurse, a better physician, and so on. Sometimes, they are surprised when they learn what their colleagues do, for example, that social workers often help families with funeral arrangements. They value such new knowledge because they know they can now use it to help families, for example, they can contact social workers as a resource when a baby dies. EPPs also show respect by explicitly expressing their appreciation for their colleagues:

> I think just showing appreciation for things helps the team. It's always easy to see something that went wrong and to focus on that. We do need to see those things that were done incorrectly and fix them so that they don't continue to happen, but I think it's also good to reinforce the things that people are doing well. So I consciously try to say, 'Good job!' or something positive, because as humans we need positive reinforcement.

Fostering a Culture of Caring

EPPs excel at fostering a culture of caring within their settings through actions that acknowledge the human responses to significant moments, events, or situations. For example, when a child dies, a candle is lit in the hospice at the start of weekly team rounds and memories are shared about the child. In all settings, EPPs notice and respond to a colleague's sense of overwhelm during exceptionally busy or stressful times by taking concrete actions, such as lending a helping hand or adjusting patient assignments whenever possible:

> Say there is an end-of-life baby coming in today and I'm going to be on for the next few days. But if I just finished working for a number of weeks with a very ill baby and it was very intense and I need a break, I might just say, 'Look, I can't go there right now.' And one of the nurses who has not had that recent experience will take the new child and be more able to be fully present with that child.

EPPs encourage debriefing sessions where team members can share perspectives and responses to morally distressing situations, such as a complicated ethical issue. Recognizing the stress of the work in their setting, some EPPs organize off-site retreat days for team members to spend a day together engaging in relaxing and fun activities. They find such days to be a real gift because they can practice some skills, learn more about—and perhaps advance—their own practice, and engage in reflection. They recognize that in their work they deal with a lot of sadness and other emotions, and that if as practitioners they are not able to sit with those emotions, then they cannot do their work. So they try to practice and live a culture of caring, though they acknowledge that sometimes they stumble.

EPPs also volunteer to help plan and/or participate in their team's social gatherings, such as celebrations or parties. Recognizing the value of maintaining optimal health, EPPs organize and encourage colleagues to attend activities such as mindfulness or meditation sessions. Once a culture of respect, inclusion, and cohesion is established, it becomes the norm and people rise to the occasion. The result is that EPPs and their team members feel cared for, empowered, reassured, and comforted, just as parents feel when they are the recipients of EPPs' acts of kindness. Finally, EPPs foster a culture of joyful caring through the passion they have for their work and by their exemplary interactions with both parents and colleagues. EPPs' *exquisite* practice, their energy and commitment as they engage with parents or colleagues, from the words they use to their physical stance to the way they use their eyes and their body, inspires their colleagues and leaves others in awe. EPPs stand out even though colleagues are doing a good job; EPPs are inspiring role models for other team members. They also contribute to a caring culture by being relaxed, generally calm, and having a sense of humor.

Parents and Teams

Parents do talk about team, but in a different way from EPPs. In many parents' minds, teams represent a group of PHCPs who share a specialized area of expertise or function, such as the neuro team, the medical team, the nursing team, the trach (respiratory) team, the mental health team, or the clinic team. Parents perceive that each team is made up of several specialists—but parents typically interact with only one person at a time and they see that person as representing a particular team. Therefore, when that person interacts well with them, that individual creates a positive impression for the entire team. The opposite is also true. Parents appreciate team functioning when individual PHCPs are competent, relaxed, and explain what they are doing and what others will be doing; the sense that their child is in good hands is very reassuring to parents.

Parents' reliance on each professional's integrity extends to their experience with teams. Teams were first designed to help coordinate care so that patients could experience a kind of collective integrity across the system. Sometimes, however, in the course of a day so many different people will come in that parents find it very overwhelming. Parents' encounters with multiple members of a team, each of whom may tell conflicting information to the parents, can break down confidence that there is a plan shared among team members and across units. Thus, parents may experience fragmentation of services: *Inconsistency of the medical team and having different people making different decisions, everyone having different opinions—that drives me bonkers.* The good news is that the culture of teamwork is a culture of interprofessional communication with constant heads-up and inquiries about what ought to be done with and for parents. EPPs base their decisions on the foundation of listening to the voices of those they serve, checking those voices against their own assumptions, and then planning care accordingly.

When a setting is focused on whole-person care or the whole family, the team composition is more likely to include the many PHCPs who are involved in the care. In addition, being committed to family-centered care, EPPs typically regard parents as members of the team and attempt to incorporate them into the team as much as possible. From the start, they get to know the family, their particular expectations and needs. The entire team looks at all the information at the same time and knows the plan. Team members work very hard to have family team meetings not only every week or more often as a child is dying but also on a regular basis with all families as both an update and a connection; so it is more natural if the child has increasing symptoms to review how things are going and to address their hopes. Parents also recognize when they are included as team members:

> We sat down with a nurse, a doctor, the whole team, everybody all together. Not just quick rounds—we actually had a discussion about my baby's care and his future care. That was probably one of the best parts, just knowing that the whole team is going to support us throughout his care.

Parents sense that they and their child are well-cared for by a team when they witness team members working together on their child's behalf:

> I met the doctor the next morning after my son's admission. They brought me a list of 17 doctors who would be on his case, so I met each one. Well, it surprised me, but it was because they wanted to know the case. They want to learn too. They work together. It's a team and even if I don't see one of them in a week, I know they're working together. So whatever's happening with my son, they're working trying to do the best for him.
>
> They are a team. I notice between them, even though I have a different nurse every day, as soon as the nurse gets out from our room, she shares the information with the other nurse in case she needs to do something else, so the other nurse knows the same information. So they are a team because everybody shares the information. That makes me feel they all know about my child. They all know what's happening here.

EPPs are aware of how alert parents are to team functioning. They understand that parents very easily can sense tension or hostility between team members. EPPs know that parents feel better when they see PHCPs working together because they feel there is a team looking out for their child. When teams are functioning well and parents feel that they and their child are well cared for, it is because people who need help are getting it and the person who is willing and able to help is being asked. When this is not happening, then resources are being underutilized and the care of children and their parents is not at its best. One EPP described teamwork as *like a patchwork quilt the way all the pieces get fitted together. It's not seamless and sometimes there's little rough tufts, but eventually it's how the care all comes together to form a blanket to hold a family.*

Challenges in Teamwork

EPPs recognize that there are challenges inherent in teamwork. They are aware that even the most optimally functioning teams encounter challenges and competing pressures from many directions, such as striving to meet children's and parents' needs and goals, managing numerous cases simultaneously, dealing with the uncertainty of CCC trajectories and outcomes, and engaging in complex problem-solving and decision-making—all while keeping in mind organizational requirements. The busy pace of work, and also a natural desire to avoid conflict, can be barriers to how teams work together, but all teams encounter conflict at times when not everyone is in agreement. EPPs wisely respond to conflict by engaging in reflection:

> When there's conflict, I know it could go back to some basic stuff within myself as a person and I'm getting buttons pushed by somebody on the team. If I'm the source of some conflict with my team member, I need to ask myself, 'What's that coming from? Is it something about what I see that they're not seeing?' Then, we should be able to talk about it. 'Is it something about my position on the team versus that person's?' I have to be ready to be open and to accept what that is about. I need to listen to my colleagues and I need to grow. I need to be ready to say, 'I'm wrong' if I'm wrong or 'Help me see what you're seeing because maybe I'm not seeing it.' So, we have to be open and respectful and ready to get past our old stuff, which hopefully we're working on in our own lives. It's about needing to grow and learn and remembering that it's not about me; it's about the family and the child and the bigger team. So I have to be open and really ready to examine myself as a person within the team or encourage my teammates to be open and reflective, willing to grow.

EPPs encourage awareness that the entire team shares a primary commitment to the best interests of the child and family, which allows members to work together to address immediate needs and set conflicts aside in order to address the immediate situation.

EPPs realize that the processing of team dynamics needs attention if members are to work together as effectively as they can. This process is not often actively facilitated in many health-care settings, but EPPs strive to create a structure for checking in on the team's health and functioning. Because of their broad worldview, EPPs are able to step back and see these types of challenges from a systems' perspective. For example, if a new program is just starting from the ground up, then EPPs want to create the opportunity for others to think about it as part of the larger system. EPPs see things as larger wholes, as complex systems, and they know that changes to the system take time.

While thinking in this way, EPPs patiently persist in keeping their eye on the overall vision of where they want to go. They know that they have to keep working at it even though sometimes they go forward a little bit and then backward; the important piece for them is to keep thinking about how to approach these new challenges. Such approaches are greatly facilitated when administrators are EPPs themselves. EPPs recognize that though teams, like themselves, are constantly evolving and changing, teams are always only a component of a larger, evolving whole. So despite believing that really good work happens in their team, EPPs recognize that the environment needs to be one in which they are still learning, because they do not know all the answers and they are just a part of the system, not all of it. Keeping their eye on their vision (worldview/values) and their commitment to authentic engagement facilitates EPPs' ability to deal with challenges beyond their individual settings to the institutional and societal challenges that are inevitable in any organization.

Further Thoughts on Setting and Teamwork Contextual Factors

We understand that there are some contextual factors that would be difficult for individuals to change. However, we do believe that at least some changes are possible. Our focus in this section is on what you as an individual can do right now as you consider your practice. We found that how well someone *fits* with their work environment can play a significant role in satisfaction with one's job and, ultimately, may contribute to a lower risk of burnout. So, it is important for you to consider the fit between your workplace and what you need to thrive. Reflect on the types of environments you have worked in, including using questions in Box 9.1. Then think about where you work now. Try to specifically identify ways in which your current context is different from other places where you have worked and then think about how well you fit in your current work environment. Now clearly identify what your ideal work environment would look like. It is not likely that you work in an ideal setting, but if there are too many discrepancies between your ideal and your current work environment, then perhaps you need to consider a change of workplace. Otherwise, you may find yourself unhappy, and your work context may negatively affect your interactions with parents and colleagues.

Whether you are able to leave your current position or not, by thinking about what EPPs do in their work settings you can consider how you could enhance *optimal teamwork*. Well-functioning teams do not just happen; they

---

Box 9.1:   Setting and Teamwork Contextual Factors—Fit With Work Environment: Questions for Consideration

- Thinking about the types of environments I have worked in, what stands out for me as being positive? What was more negative?
- As I ponder my past experiences, do I see a fit or a disconnect between my values and those settings? Did a lack of fit perhaps make me consider finding another job?
- What, if any, meaning do I find in the work I do currently?
- Does the work I do in my current workplace reflect my values? How?
- How well do I fit with my current environment?
- What do I want in a work environment? What would my ideal work environment look like?
- Is there a good fit between what I want and what I have in my current environment?

---

require effort. Think about your current team, what you like about it, and who is included (see Box 9.2). We learned a lot from drawing the diagrams of communication flow within teams. Try drawing your own diagram of your perception of how communication flows within your team, as well as between your team and other teams. What insights did you gain from this exercise? You also can learn a lot about teamwork by observing team meetings or conferences. Think back to a recent team meeting for insights on how your team functions. For example, reflect on who was present and who was missing. Did the presence or absence of people affect the decisions that were made? Having a *safe environment* is important for optimal teamwork. Consider how safety is facilitated in your team meetings (see Box 9.2). In an optimally functioning team, there is recognition of everyone's contribution. Think about what happens within your setting that facilitates open conversation about PHCPs' experiences at work and consider how you can contribute to making this type of conversation happen by creating a safe and caring environment in which people feel welcome and not judged.

You can also learn from observing the physical environment. For example, Betty once visited a children's hospital where a plaque at the front door stated: "The physicians and staff welcome you." She appreciated the intention of hospitality, but at the same time the wording clearly implied that the physicians were in a group separate from all other staff, which is not exactly the most positive message about teamwork. You might look to see how team or teamwork is described on your institution's website. What

Box 9.2:   Setting and Teamwork Contextual Factors—Optimal Teamwork: Questions for Consideration

- What do I like when working with my team?
- What stands out for me as being especially important?
- Who are particular colleagues I have learned from?
- What insights have I gained by observing and listening to colleagues?
- Who does my team include?
- What do I appreciate as being unique about my workplace?
- What gives me pride in the teamwork within my setting?

Team Meetings

- When reflecting on a recent team meeting, who was present, and who do I think was missing? Did the presence or absence of people affect the decisions that were made?
- What was the nature of the discussion—for example, did it focus only on giving factual information (such as a report), or was there space for asking questions, clarifying comments, and sharing emotions?

Safe Environments

- How is respect demonstrated by me and my colleagues?
- If there are any problematic behaviors, how are they handled and by whom?
- How do I see team members being acknowledged and listened to, or not?

Describing Team or Teamwork

- In my workplace, is one discipline consistently described as the leader of the team?
- How, if at all, are other disciplines mentioned?
- Can I think of additional, more inclusive ways for my institution to describe team and teamwork? If so, who are the people who have the power to make changes, the people I can then take my ideas to?
- What are my plans for effecting change if needed?

underlying messages do those descriptions give? Do they need to change? There are multiple ways that you and your colleagues can attempt to influence what happens in your setting. Think about one thing you tried to change in your setting. What happened? Were you successful or not? What did you learn from this experience so that you can be (more) successful the next time?

Collaboration is an essential feature of effective teamwork. But *challenges in teamwork* can arise for a variety of reasons, for example, differences in understanding disciplinary roles, in professional values and behaviors, in setting priorities, in levels of power, and in policies and procedures. Reflect on a time when there was a challenge within your team and consider how challenges are handled by your team (see Box 9.3). Letting problems continue eventually leads to a breakdown in teamwork, so it is important that you learn how to be an effective team member who is able to promote high-quality team functioning. Think about a specific colleague you view as someone who tries to find common ground and who works effectively to maintain harmony in the team. Consider what you might learn from that person to enhance your own practice. If you are unsure of what your colleagues actually do in their jobs, be creative in thinking about what you might do to ensure you understand your colleagues' roles and the work they do.

Being a leader in your setting does not necessarily mean that you have to hold a formal leadership role, such as a unit manager, though if you do have a formal role, then being an EPP is likely to make you an exemplary leader. *Informal leadership* skills and contributions also can help optimize team functioning, and informal leaders are role models for colleagues. A strong informal leader can transform the workplace culture and have a positive effect on the experiences of people working in the setting. Informal leaders are good at building relationships with just about anybody; so they are inclusive. They know how things work within their unit and their institution, which means they are great people to ask about the history of your workplace and the unspoken rules that you know exist and are afraid of inadvertently breaking.

You will recognize informal leaders because they are the ones who happily share their knowledge with others and do not look for or expect any payback. They also know what things are worth fighting for versus those that are not; so when you are uncertain about speaking out about something, they can provide an excellent listening ear and some wise advice. Finally, informal leaders typically are not afraid to try something new, and they are likely to be the early adopters of new tools and technologies; they do not sit back and wait until others have taken the first steps. Consider how these characteristics of informal leaders fit with your worldview, values, and sense of commitment (see Box 9.3). Once you identify your own leadership strengths and areas for improvement, you can build on those strengths and deliberately work on improving in other areas.

In this chapter, we have discussed the group of factors that is particular to the immediate work environment, that is, setting and teamwork. But there is another group of factors that also can affect PHCPs' ability to practice optimally. In the next chapter, we will discuss this second group of

---

Box 9.3: Setting and Teamwork Contextual Factors—Challenges in Teamwork, Informal Leadership: Questions for Consideration

Challenges in Teamwork

- When reflecting on a recent challenge within my team, do I think the challenge was dealt with or ignored?
- How effective was the response (or lack thereof) to this challenge?
- In general, how well does my team handle differences?
- When thinking about colleagues who I believe try to find common ground and work effectively to maintain harmony in the team, what actions do I see them taking? What words do they use? What else do I see as being important in how they manage differences within the team?
- What could I learn from those colleagues to help me enhance how I should respond to differences or contribute to finding common ground?
- How can I learn more about various disciplinary perspectives?
- How can I find a way of organizing presentations by colleagues to each other? Or of spending time shadowing a colleague for even short periods of time?

Informal Leadership

- How do I recognize informal leaders?
- How do informal leaders inspire me to be an informal leader?
- How do I think others would characterize my current influence as a leader?
- How would I characterize my influence?

---

contextual factors that encompasses the broader environment—the institution and society.

Note

1. Primary nursing is a model of nursing care delivery that assigns a single nurse or small group of nurses to provide the majority of a patient's care during their inpatient hospital admission. The primary nurse or nurses receive preferential assignment to the patient, that is, when the nurse is working they will care for the patient for whom they are designated as primary. The primary nurse may communicate with other nurses caring for the patient to ensure that those nurses are up to date on the patient's plan of care, and the primary nurse may also be responsible for attending care conferences

or family meetings to help support and/or represent the patient or family. The goal of primary nursing is to provide continuity of nursing care across the hospital admission, which may become particularly relevant for patients who experience a long length of stay (Manthey, 2002).

References

Manthey, M. (2002). *The practice of primary nursing* (2nd ed.). Springer Publishing.
Youngwerth, J., & Twaddle, M. (2011). Cultures of interdisciplinary teams: How to foster good dynamics. *Journal of Palliative Medicine, 14*(5), 650–654. http://doi.org/10.1089/jpm.2010.0395

10 Institutional and Societal Contextual Factors

Well, I think the big scheme is important. Going to that conference was good for me because I got to see the bigger picture stuff that, day-to-day, I don't see here. All those meetings, hearing how they're trying to put pediatric palliative care in words on paper so that government and potential donors will even acknowledge that pediatric palliative care exists in society. And, then how some government money may filter down to individual places like here. If our budget falls apart, that affects everything. That's pretty awesome because those meetings are the first step in a huge number of steps to make things better here. Of course, it all fits together and affects what I do. It's all the concept of 'How aware are we of our environment?' If you're not paying attention to what's around you, how will you pay attention to the families, and to yourself?

As highlighted in Chapter 9, the setting, teamwork, institutional context, and broader society in which PHCPs work all affect their ability to practice to their potential. These factors can either enhance or constrain practice. We discussed the immediate set of factors, setting and teamwork, in Chapter 9 and in this chapter we focus on the second group of factors that encompass the broader environment, that is, the institutional setting, including leadership at the unit and institutional levels, and the broader society in which PHCPs work.

Institutional Factors

Our study encompassed settings from three institutions that provide specialized care for neonates, children, and/or adolescents—populations that present a particularly unique feature to the institutional context of interactions because age is a constant consideration. Four important institutional factors were evident: (1) The nuances of *Serving a Pediatric Population*, (2) the *Relative Richness of Pediatric Funding and Resources*, (3) the *Impact of Policies and Procedures* on delivery of pediatric care, and (4) the *Quality of Leadership at Institutional and Setting Levels*.

Serving a Pediatric Population

A child's age necessitates attention in every aspect of the institution, for example, having appropriate-sized equipment, the medications required

DOI: 10.4324/9780429352393-10

for children's diagnoses, child-sized doses of these medications, and policies and procedures that take into account both the children and their families, including the fact that many families travel long distances to these institutions that are generally regional in scope. Such policies and procedures can also be affected by systemic societal issues, such as sexism, that filter through to the institution. For example, the assumption often is that the mother is the primary caregiver, but fathers often want to be included and involved in the care, decisions, and treatment of their children. Fathers, therefore, sometimes feel left out, sidelined, or marginalized. For example, the physical setup may focus more on mothers, rightly so at times such as the pump room in the NICU. But even when infants are bottle-fed, sometimes fathers need to remind others that they too can participate in feeding their infant.

It also is essential that caregivers understand children's physical, cognitive, and psychosocial development, as well as each child's particular health-care needs. EPPs are at ease with children. They understand that youngsters are sometimes boisterous and other times silent, but always inquisitive. EPPs realize that caring for groups of children can be rather chaotic, as anyone who has visited daycare centers, classrooms, playgrounds, or gatherings of youth sports teams will know. EPPs feel comfortable interacting with children, often acting a bit silly with them, and they remain calm in the face of what may seem to others like chaos. EPPs recognize that they have a natural rapport with infants, children, and/or adolescents and intentionally choose to work with them, often immediately after their initial professional education. Something as relatively simple as having a high tolerance for children crying and seeing it as a challenge that needs a solution rather than as upsetting could be an impetus to enter the pediatric field. EPPs' worldview includes perceiving children not as tiny adults, but as human beings filled with developmental potential, and they treasure the opportunity to see the world from the child's perspective.

But caring for ill children presents numerous challenges. When children with complex, chronic, and potentially life-threatening conditions (CCCs) are ill, their situation can be precarious. Rare childhood conditions are often difficult to diagnose, and irregular disease trajectories mean that uncertainty about medical prognostication and day-to-day life is inevitable. Children's reactions to treatments are variable and their physiological status can change rapidly. Because some patients are too young to talk, keen assessment skills and reliance on knowledgeable intuition are required. EPPs undoubtedly have had to perfect their style of history taking, assessment skills, and clinical care. Furthermore, when children are seriously ill their all-round vulnerability— and that of their parents—is pronounced; EPPs acknowledge that vulnerability. They ensure they have a wide-ranging knowledge base and their systems' perspective means that their care embraces the whole family.

Institutions that care for children are typically committed to advancing children's health and health care. All three of our study institutions are affiliated with nearby educational institutions; thus, a great deal of teaching, research, and academic-related work is woven into the daily lives of PHCPs in these settings, even though their primary responsibilities may be clinical, frontline services for children, women, and families. EPPs enjoy the range of possibilities and eagerly take on the mentoring of new and inexperienced PHCPs, as well as students. They also are supportive of research, not just because it is required as part of their position but because they are eager to learn and to contribute to developing and improving initiatives that will advance knowledge about children's health.

Relative Richness in Pediatric Funding and Resources

Similar to settings that treat adults, pediatric institutions typically receive a large part of their funding from government sources, even in the US with its mainly private insurance system. Therefore, they are vulnerable to the vagaries of decisions made by the politicians who are in charge of setting priorities. When the government changes, then funding can be jeopardized or enhanced depending on the new list of priorities. But unlike adult facilities, specializing in serving children often has the advantage of facilitating the fund-raising that is a necessary resource for supporting several aspects of an institution, for example, equipment or research. Concern about campaigns that exploit children with little bald heads or newborns hooked up to monstrous equipment that seems to dwarf such helpless little souls is sometimes a challenge for PHCPs and fundraisers. But generally, such photographs and accompanying stories are sensitively used and are effective; people love to give money to children's causes.

Successful fund-raising is the reason that many PHCPs acknowledge they have access to a range of resources in their setting. EPPs in particular express their gratitude for such resources and are actively involved in some fund-raising efforts. Similarly, many parents express appreciation for the services that are available: *The children's hospital is a much more caring place and personal place than adult acute facilities where parents go for treatment.*

Despite the extra funding, some resource limitations, for example, crowded physical space and outdated equipment, are problematic for both parents and PHCPs. But some PHCPs, particularly EPPs, are able to be more creative than others in finding solutions. EPPs believe that resource issues are important for the way people deal with them—whether they perceive the glass as half-full or half-empty, whether or not they are able to manage with what is available, and whether or not they are frustrated and even angry with a lack of facilities, equipment, or funding. EPPs remain consistently appreciative of institutional resources and when they see a need for potential change, they strive to make it known, suggest remedies, and foster the desired change.

Impact of Policies and Procedures

Institutional culture, policies, and procedures have an impact on how people feel about their place in the system and can support, or not, parents and

PHCPs alike. They should be helpful, guide the workflow, and both assist and support everyone. However, when institutional policies become bureaucratic or dogmatic, or when people disagree with them, then they become a source of tension. When menacing possibilities (Frank, 2004) originate at the institutional level, for example, the possibility of reduced funding, staff cuts, or discontinuing programs, settings are affected and clinicians feel the angst. EPPs acknowledge that their institutions go through ups and downs, with quite troubled times because of finances or changes in structure, for example, at the management or board levels. But EPPs also know that seeing a bigger picture helps with such stressors. So when a program first opens, for example, they think of it in developmental terms, as a baby. New initiatives are going to take baby steps, then toddler steps, and they are going to fall down so that they can get up again to grow. Then they go into the youth phase and the adult phase of growth. Understanding the bigger picture helps EPPs make sense of and be more tolerant of what is happening.

Institutional flexibility with policies that optimize PHCPs' work arrangements enhances PHCPs' happiness and potential for engaging in exemplary interactions at all levels of the institution. Policies that, for example, accommodate different work patterns or schedules, allow two part-time people to share one position, or offer leaves of absence as an option to support self-care set a tone of caring for others. A practice of strategically hiring only people who fit the particular position rather than just filling a position for the sake of expediency contributes to optimal functioning. A structure that allows for examining practices to evaluate whether something is a time-honored routine or if there is a more effective way of doing things to achieve the institution's larger purpose shows a willingness to change as needed. Such flexibility is based upon administrators, managers, and all health-care workers understanding each other's roles, challenges, and contributions to the institution's goal of providing optimal care to children and their families.

Working with seriously ill children means the work environment is characterized by constant change requiring immediate attention. Dealing with such adjustments is not usually problematic for PHCPs, particularly for EPPs who find the unanticipated nature of their work—the planning for multiple eventualities—challenging and even exciting. EPPs enjoy situations that keep them busy, challenged, and engaged, but not overloaded or stressed. They are flexible, ready for whatever happens, and able to act accordingly. The typical mixture of busy/chaotic and quiet days appeals to EPPs who enjoy working with these populations because the variety of issues they face, for example, acute, end-of-life, bereavement, grief, trauma, and shock issues, all compound the challenges. EPPs seem to thrive in their constantly changing environment.

At the same time, constantly dealing with challenges in pediatric settings and the ever-increasing institutional expectations to do more in less time sometimes leaves PHCPs feeling that they lack enough time to spend with the children and their parents. The combination of ever-increasing caseloads, sicker patients with increasing complexity, being short-staffed, and having excessive administrative tasks on top of their clinical responsibilities may also result in less time for debriefing with colleagues or for personal reflection. EPPs respond to similar perceptions by stepping back, even momentarily, when they recognize that they are feeling overwhelmed or frustrated and they acknowledge the value of tending to their own needs—both inside and outside of work—to ensure they remain present and fully engaged in their practice. Moreover, EPPs' inclusive worldview allows them to step back and see the situation from a systems perspective, so they can envision what else could be done. Their wide-angle lens allows them to be either familiar with or eager to discover available resources and then utilize them to help children and their parents.

Leadership at Institutional and Setting Levels

Leadership at every level, but particularly at the institutional and setting levels for our purposes in this chapter, is instrumental in creating a caring environment that best promotes human-to-human interaction for PHCPs and families alike. When the institutional culture is one in which everyone—administrators, managers, clinicians, and staff—feel as if they are in it together and striving for a common goal, then they perceive that they are all part of the same community or team. Leaders who interact in similar ways to EPPs recognize that the pressures of administrative and clinical demands are felt by everyone, so they will say, *We need to ask the staff* or *We need to go back and ask the parents.* Then the staff, clinicians, and parents can share their concerns, suggestions, experiences, thoughts, and ideas with the administrators and managers. Consequently, communication flows freely among all participants.

These types of administrators understand that before they initiate a project they first need to pay attention to those who may be involved. They are very mindful about how to approach projects and they realize that understanding what they are trying to change also affects how the improvement happens. They take into consideration whether they need to build groups that are sustainable over time or if they want a group that just swoops in, fixes the problem, and comes back out again. These administrators acknowledge existing groups, so rather than just starting a new project, they first determine if they can filter work to an existing group and then provide resources to help make the needed change happen.

At the setting level, EPP leaders are available to offer feedback not only when things go wrong but also when they go well. Such leaders are pivotal in promoting a positive environment. Though thoughtful responses take time and careful planning, and occur within a challenging aspect of today's world, that is, the widespread sense of too much to do and too little time, EPPs as clinicians and as leaders make time to mindfully focus on the moment and, thus, help to create a culture of openhearted compassion and caring.

Societal Factors

Just as individuals work within teams in settings located in institutions, institutions also exist within the broader context of society. Societal developments can challenge not only institutional resources and expectations for settings but also individual clinicians and their teams. Three societal factors stood out in our analysis: (1) The *Corporatization of Health Care*, (2) *Working in a Technological World*, and (3) *Societal Attitudes Toward Death*.

Corporatization of Health Care

The contexts within which PHCPs work—setting, institution, society—are structured according to values, and those values determine what is given priority and worth. Indeed, the health care world seems to be increasingly guided by disease/treatment, not the search for well-being, and by the business model of care that reflects nearly every realm of human activity now being called an industry, for example, the health-care industry, the education industry, the movie industry, and the banking industry. As the cost and complexity of health care have increased over time, so too have efforts to reduce expenses and introduce standardization using principles from corporate industries. The corporatization of health care has shifted attention away from the PHCP–patient–parent relationship and placed focus on depersonalized mass production and the commodity–consumer relationship, with a corresponding emphasis on measurement and productivity. Consequently, very precise ratings exist for safety and for whether or not the rules and regulations are followed. The number of procedures PHCPs can do are counted and PHCPs are congratulated for how adeptly and quickly they do them. But there are no good metrics for a setting's success in achieving excellence in interaction; there is no way of measuring what is involved in listening to a parent or to a colleague in distress.

This business model of care shapes how in their practice PHCPs relate to others and respond in their interactions. As practitioners, they end up feeling responsible for many things on their to-do lists, but they also may feel constrained in fulfilling their responsibilities to parents as human beings: *As we get busier, we sacrifice the stuff of figuring out what people need and making sure that those needs are being met. We have to be careful that we watch that; it's a big issue.* EPPs, however, have some immunity to such outcomes because their worldview and commitment to authentic engagement sustains them. It is important to note that EPPs say it is not that they sustain their commitment; rather, they are sustained by their commitment to being authentic with others.

Working in a Technological World

Technological developments in health care have saved innumerable lives and are continuously improving quality of life, but such developments also have had a profound impact on nearly all processes and practices for PHCPs. For example, children with various CCCs are living longer and may present with acute illness that requires intensive treatment, making a difference for the PHCPs who care for them at the bedside: *You have to do more maintaining of procedures, e.g., intrathecal catheters and pumps that we have not used before. As long as they are working, it's okay. We're pretty good at helping each other out.* We found, however, that whereas all clinicians have to learn to manage increasingly complicated equipment, EPPs tend to find a positive in the situation:

> While checking the pump, you can chat to the patient or the parent, enhance rapport. So yes and no, the new technologies add to our workload, and it's stressful when it's new, but as long as you can be adaptable with it you're okay. For example, you can say to yourself, 'I have to be in here giving blood, I have to sit here for the first 15 minutes of blood going through. What a great opportunity! I'm going to hang out with this family for 15 minutes!'

Global expansion in the realm of information and communication technology, such as telehealth, might link PHCPs with each other and also connect them with patients, but PHCPs complain that the level of complexity and the level of information and the context in which they are practicing have exploded. As long as internet connectivity is available, technology is especially useful in enhancing efficiency within institutions, across institutions, and in more rural areas and locations that lack facilities and/or specialists. With such developments as the electronic health record (EHR) though, EPPs note that many problems still need to be worked out. They had thought that computerized charts would help, but the reality is that they still have to do everything on paper as well so that the EHR just duplicates everything. Moreover, these systems require that extensive amounts of data are inputted into central, digitized systems. Doing so takes considerable time for clinicians who already have heavy workloads.

A frequent lament by all PHCPs, including EPPs, is about the wave of bureaucracy, an artifact of health-care corporatization, they face every day. A common sentiment is the idea that PHCPs are drowning in paperwork. EPPs manage their paperwork fairly well, but when administrative tasks that must be done as part of their work are exceeded by what they see as bureaucratic demands or excess bureaucracy, such as when a request to make a simple change requires many levels of time-consuming approval or when EPPs perceive administrative demands as interfering with their clinical decision-making, they experience what we have named *bureaucratic fatigue*. EPPs see themselves as being able to make changes in the system, but even they can be discouraged by what seems like more and more and more forms to complete, boxes to check, and reports to write. Their frustration is apparently not unique to participants in our study as similar findings have been described in the results of an investigative inquiry into the success of EHRs (Fry & Schulte, 2019) in which the authors concluded that EHRs still result in a patchwork of disconnected systems that cause multiple problems for PHCPs while enriching the companies that sell EHR systems.

Another result of the increased use of technology, driven in part by an increase in litigation, has been societal pressure for greater regulation of such systems. Therefore, external accrediting bodies have become common and they require more and more information-gathering for purposes such as provider accountability and budgetary rationale/expenditure. This information-gathering creates still more additional work for PHCPs to complete, contributing to the sense that they are being pulled away from patient care responsibilities and the meaningful work they want to be doing.

Despite these challenges, EPPs' worldview enables them to remain focused on the positive benefits of enhanced technology and the ways in which they can work to overcome or counteract the challenges that changing technologies bring. EPPs' ability to see the positive in situations enables them to persist in learning more about technological advancements and keeping alive their hope that technology will have a positive impact on not just improving efficiency but also on preserving and enhancing the human aspects of health care.

Societal Attitudes Toward Death

A prevailing attitude within Westernized societies is that serious illness should not strike children; children dying is against the natural order. But it is not just the death of children that arouses discomfort within society. Sociologists suggest that modern societies sequester or push death to the edges of society or at least out of public view and discourse. Hospitals are perceived as places where death is to be conquered or, when unable to be conquered, to be hidden away (Papadatou, 2009). As members of the broader society, PHCPs who care for children with CCCs regularly face end-of-life situations and are also influenced by these societal attitudes. Our participants in oncology and the NICU acknowledged that people very seldom talk about death on their units. When the priority is to extend life, sacrificing the quality of a child's existence now by putting them into intensive care, performing surgery, or providing chemotherapy offers the chance of gaining time later. In hospice, it is expected that children will die, so the priority is to offer the fullest possible lives right now; death is a recurring topic of gentle conversation.

In intensive and acute care settings, the unrelenting pace of work may contribute to suppressing conversations about death: *The pace, along with the stress of parents whose baby might die, results in emotional strain that means it can be a struggle to get to talk to parents.* Similar to the general population, parents do not typically want to talk about death, especially their own child's death, but these parents need PHCPs who are comfortable conversing about death. Yet, these conversations can be difficult even for some EPPs. PHCPs can have a hard time with transitioning from providing intensive care where they are focused on curing to providing or transferring to palliative care. Some see it as a *total shift* and perhaps a failure of the nature of what they are meant to do, although others are getting more comfortable with the idea that *death is a normal part of life; it is not wrong to accept that it's okay to let children die when they cannot recover.*

It is very difficult even for EPPs when they have known a family for a long time and now have to tell the parents that their child is going to die. The pressures of a chaotic environment also mean fewer opportunities for PHCPs to meet and talk with one another, precluding the personal and professional renewal that might happen during debriefing. Sometimes, the pace is so fast that patients die and PHCPs do not have time to slow down because in half an hour there is another sick baby. It is traumatic for PHCPs when they are expected to go back to business without a break as soon as the child's body leaves the unit.

How PHCPs deal with death stems also from societal attitudes about how, or if, the topic of death is incorporated into educational curricula. Across settings, our participants noted that as students in their respective healthcare programs, or even as young clinicians, they received little preparation for dealing with death and grief nor were they told where or how to get support in their clinical roles as professionals. Over and over they are taught technical skills, for example, how to insert an IV, but they are not prepared for the angry outbursts of parents who are in pain about their child's impending death. They are not taught how to talk to grieving parents, or how not to talk to them. Even in their clinical workplaces, education about death, dying, and bereavement is limited, if offered at all. Perhaps there will be a short talk and some pamphlets will be handed out but typically there is no coordinated or ongoing effort to educate about death. Some PHCPs are reluctant to talk about death because they think of death as a failure. But others eventually learn through experience that death is not necessarily failure—there are a lot of things worse than death. But they usually had to learn that all on their own.

EPPs, although aware of society's disinclination to discuss death or acknowledge grief, are distinguished from other PHCPs by their personal attitudes and comfort with death. Their worldview encompasses the idea that death is part of life for everyone. They understand that life is beautiful but also difficult and that even children get sick and die. Some EPPs choose to work in palliative care because they know that however people arrive at death, it happens to everyone. These EPPs want to look at death directly as a way to make it as meaningful, as reconciling, and as beautiful a remembrance as possible for families. Feeling comfortable with the idea of death is requisite to EPPs' understanding of parents' grief:

> You're going to see the worst in everybody. Their child is dying, so why should we expect them to be normal and happy and always have good conversations with others? Each member of a couple grieves differently, taking turns at being more together or losing it but it might be the opposite another time. Like all people, we need to trust that we're going through a process, that we're all grieving in different ways and that's normal grief.

Societal attitudes about what is normal grief also come into play. EPPs appreciate that in many cultures grief is much more outwardly expressed than is typical in North American society: *We do value holding it in and I've heard judgment placed on others as being hysterical when their wailing is actually not in any way out of their norm.* Societal attitudes also have a practical impact, for example, the general public is more eager to donate to life-saving projects rather than to bereavement programs that are reminders of death. In response, EPPs often creatively engage in designing such programs themselves. For example, they lead grief support groups or make follow-up phone calls to bereaved families.

EPPs are aware that death is inherent in their work. They believe that the dying, grief, and loss aspects of what they do are extremely important. As clinicians, they experience many losses but they embrace that reality and do not pull away. EPPs view it as an honor to be on this journey with families and they take their role very seriously. EPPs also believe that all clinicians, especially in settings caring for children with CCCs, must be prepared to respond to issues surrounding death because PHCPs can never know if when a child's parents leave the room the child will ask if they are dying. Or if a parent will ask directly about their child dying. EPPs are aware that learning how to interact with these children and parents is possible, but it is a long process that should start much earlier in life and especially in education programs. They also understand that they will use that learning not just at work but also in their personal lives.

To help themselves and their colleagues with grief, EPPs actively participate in and encourage debriefing sessions, consult with chaplains and social workers who are particularly skilled in containing emotion, sit for a while with one another to share the burden of grief, or develop rituals. They realize that such activities may not be how people generally think about health care in North American society—these activities may be something that are considered extra, but maybe not essential. However, EPPs believe that how PHCPs deal with death and grief is essential to their humanity, to who they are as human beings.

Further Thoughts on Institutional and Societal Contextual Factors

We understand that the institutional and societal contextual factors can be difficult for individuals to change. However, we do believe that there are actions individuals can take, such as pushing back against the corporatization of health care and educating the broader population about death and dying.

EPPs were aware of the increasing shift toward *corporatization* and the accompanying standardization of processes, some of which worked counter to the goal of providing individualized patient and family-centered care. They also recognized the roles they could play in helping to counterbalance the corporate feel of health care. Consider how you can effect change if you feel that care delivery is becoming depersonalized and/or focused on productivity rather than human connection (see Box 10.1 for questions to think about). Perhaps you could raise the topic at a unit staff meeting or an institutional townhall. You might consider joining a committee that is focused on understanding and improving the patient/family experience of care, or one where you can work to include the voice of the patient/family in decision-making about institutional processes. Using patient/family feedback to help improve the quality of care your team delivers might be another approach. Similarly, it is important to understand clinicians' experience of the work environment. Consider how you could use employee engagement surveys to improve the work experience for team members. If you or other members of your team are feeling frustrated with the level of depersonalization and the focus on measurement and productivity, you might advocate for changes to the work environment that support humanistic, personalized care delivery, recognition of the value of individual team members, and measurement of the things that matter, such as patient/family experience and team member satisfaction with how care is being delivered.

Similarly, advocacy for an optimal clinical work environment might include a focus on appropriate use of *technology*. You might consider joining the hospital's clinical documentation committee to help guide how, when, and for what purpose updates are made to the EHR and to identify and advocate for ways to streamline documentation and better connect existing systems. Many hospitals also have a value analysis committee to review the use of supplies and equipment deployed to clinical areas, and these committees can benefit from the perspectives of clinicians who are using the equipment in practice.

Our study took place within the context of children with life-threatening conditions. Yet we realized that despite the relatively high numbers of infants who die annually in the NICU and the percentage of children with cancer who do not survive, *death* was not a topic that came up in our conversations with clinicians in those areas without explicit prompting. On the other hand, clinicians in hospice were much more open about death and dying. Moreover, across settings, it was the EPPs who seemed most

Box 10.1: Institutional and Societal Contextual Factors: Questions for Consideration

Institutional

- When thinking about a time I felt that care delivery was becoming depersonalized and/or focused on productivity rather than human connection, what avenues were available to me to raise concerns? How could I have used those avenues? What about in the future?
- How can I use my professional voice to advocate for authentic, relationship-based care delivery in my setting?
- In my work area, do we regularly review and discuss patient/family satisfaction surveys or other sources of data about the patient/family experience?
- How might I work to incorporate patient/family feedback into plans for improving the quality of care my team delivers?
- Does my organization conduct employee engagement surveys? How are these data used to improve the work experience for team members?
- How might I or other members of my team advocate for changes to the work environment that support what we view as being important?
- What mechanisms exist for me to provide feedback on charting in the EHR or on the use of equipment in clinical areas?

Societal: Death and Dying

- What do I think is the relationship between my worldview and my beliefs about death?
- Have I thought much about death and dying? What about my own death: Do I spend any time pondering my death?
- What feelings do I have about death and dying as a concept, for example, uncomfortable, afraid, open, curious, and so on?
- How are my attitudes toward death linked to the ways in which I interacted with previous dying patients and their parents? How I dealt with the parents' reactions?
- If I have not yet had such an experience, would I know what to do and what to say?
- What gaps in knowledge and skills do I have that might contribute to less than fulfilling interactions? What are my plans for closing those gaps?

comfortable acknowledging death and who, though they valued curing illness when they could, realized that the need to cure can get in the way of an equally important goal: Helping children and families navigate the death and dying process. If you want to become an EPP or continue to improve your current practice as an EPP, then you also need to consider your beliefs about death and dying, as well as how you interact with children, families, and colleagues when a child has a life-threatening condition and/or is nearing death.

It is their worldview and values that guide EPPs in their approach to caring for dying children and the children's parents. They refine their approach and enhance their own growth through maturational learning and reflection, as well as by engaging in self-care. Consider your own attitudes toward death and use the relevant questions in Box 10.1 to prompt your reflections. As you reflect on death and dying as a concept, document how you feel, for example, uncomfortable, afraid, open, and curious. Then think back to an experience when you had to deal with the dying and death of an infant, child, or adolescent. As you remember the experience both emotionally and intellectually, can you see how your attitudes toward death are linked to the ways in which you interacted with that patient and their parents, and with how you dealt with the parents' reactions? If you have not yet had such an experience, then instead just imagine what you might do in the situation. Would you know what to do and what to say? Check in with your body and learn how you feel, even in your imagination. You should be able to identify what makes you uncomfortable, which might lead to you shying away from fully interacting with these children and their families, and also what gaps in knowledge you have that might also contribute to less than fulfilling interactions.

Whether you are experienced or not with talking about death and dying and whether you feel comfortable or not, there are always things you can learn to enhance your knowledge and skills. Consider who might be a good person in your setting to seek guidance from, to discuss your questions and concerns with. Look for workshops, conference, and books/articles to attend/read so you can increase your knowledge. Seek out experiences in which you can work with someone who is good at death and dying so you can learn through those experiential experiences. Finally, consider how you can share with the wider world what you have learned so you can help address the general societal approach of remaining silent about death.

As we reach the end of Chapter 10, we reflect on how so far in this book we have laid out our model and offered suggestions about how PHCPs can use the various components to optimize their practice. In the next chapter, we will discuss the *output* of our windmill model and identify outcomes for parents and EPPs that are associated with practicing in a way that fits our model.

References

Frank, A. (2004). *The renewal of generosity: Illness, medicine and how to live.* University of Chicago Press.

Fry, E., & Schulte, F. (2019, March 18). Death by a thousand clicks: Where electronic health records went wrong. *Fortune Magazine.* https://fortune.com/longform/medical-records/

Papadatou, D. (2009). *In the face of death: Professionals who care for the dying and the bereaved.* Springer Publishing.

11 Output From Exemplary Interaction

A Milieu of Mattering

There are so many facets to the milieu. The output of water in the windmill is life-giving, nurturing. So is the milieu of mattering—but it is also give and take. Both people feel that something meaningful has happened. It's more than just feeling that you've done a good job—it's connection.

Any serious, life-threatening condition in children is an overwhelming experience for their parents. Of utmost importance to such parents is how PHCPs interact with them during every encounter. Throughout this book, we have used the views of both pediatric providers and parents to describe the many components that contribute to exemplary interactions, that is, interactions with PHCPs who are perceived by parents as excellent and whom we describe as EPPs. We have highlighted the responses of parents to each facet of EPP interactions, as well as the responses of the EPPs themselves. Based on our analysis of those many responses, we now address the final component of our model—the overall result of exemplary interactions.

When a prairie windmill is working effectively, the shaft triggers the mechanism for pumping out ground water that sustains livestock, grain crops, and vegetation, as well as the people who live on arid prairie plains. Similarly, guided by their worldview/values and commitment to authentic engagement, EPPs' enactment of the process of attuning (the basic social process within our grounded theory study) triggers the development of relationship with parents (and others). In Chapter 8, we noted the importance of relationship as being central to exemplary interaction; but it is only one component. The coming together of all components of the model creates (or pumps out) the milieu that optimally sustains not only parents during a time of extreme duress but also the EPPs themselves in the work that they do.

Milieu

Milieu, as a concept, applies especially to the social surroundings of a person or group of persons. It is akin to the concept of social climate based on the

DOI: 10.4324/9780429352393-11

thinking and research of Dr. Rudolf Moos in the 1970s. Social climate refers to how people tend to perceive the social ambience at a given time and how they perceive it affects them. Milieu, therefore, is rooted in perception (How I see the way things are done, How people treat each other around here, or How this place makes me feel) and refers to the way that social environments, like people, have unique personalities.

The personality of the milieu between EPPs and parents evolves from EPPs enacting the process of attuning that we have described in previous chapters. Attuning leads to a milieu of mattering. In this milieu, both parents and EPPs feel that they and their concerns matter to each other and that neither is left alone to face the challenges of caring for children with CCCs. Parents feel that they and those who matter most to them—their children—are treated with respect and with their human dignity intact. EPPs feel similarly respected and valued by parents. In this milieu, both EPPs and parents perceive a sense of cohesion, a sense of being united by and committed to common interests that matter—providing the best possible care to the children. Both EPPs and parents experience a sense of interconnectedness and of belonging, a feeling that they are in it together. A sense of openness permits EPPs and parents to honestly share information and to feel safe and comfortable in speaking out about what matters to them without fear of recrimination. A sense of expressiveness predisposes EPPs and parents to willingly share a wide range of thoughts, feelings, and concerns about what matters. In this milieu, parents are satisfied with and grateful for the care they receive from EPPs who treat them not just as parents but as persons in their own right. Parents feel that EPPs relate to them as fellow human beings, as companions in dealing with one of life's most challenging experiences. Importantly, in this milieu parents freely express their appreciation to the EPPs; thus, EPPs feel valued by the parents. Both EPPs and parents feel that they are making a difference in the lives of one another. Further, while working within their team to make a difference in the lives of families, EPPs engage in exemplary interactions with their colleagues and contribute to team members feeling that they too belong and matter to each other.

This milieu of mattering, occurring when all the components of attuning come together, is represented by the windmill's output of a strong spray of water that diffuses widely and nourishes the potentially arid landscape of caring for children with CCCs. When EPPs interact according to the model (see Figure 2.2 in Chapter 2), an optimal milieu of mattering is created. Of course, all PHCP interactions with parents result in a milieu, but when PHCP interactions include only some components of the model, the milieu is of less benefit in terms of mattering. Such a milieu is less nourishing and, in our metaphor, would be illustrated by a lighter, less diffuse spray of water. The EPP–parent interpersonal milieu of mattering serves as a model for other PHCPs who observe the interaction and, thus, the milieu of mattering extends into the setting as a strong spray of water spurting further from the windmill. For example, recall how the *exquisite* style of an EPP whose connection with each parent is obvious to others inspires PHCPs to learn from and follow that EPP's approach.

Guided by their broad systems perspective, EPPs also work toward making a difference both in their institutions (institutional mattering) and beyond (societal mattering). As a result, EPPs feel like they matter at work and that they contribute to something that matters to society. Although the spray is misty at that distance, it is still effective in contributing to a milieu of mattering, which is important because the psychosocial environment that pervades health-care institutions can make people feel that they do or do not matter. The spray also showers the windmill itself, thus illustrating how the output is part of the cycle that nourishes each EPP's desire and capacity to continue practicing according to the model of exemplary interaction.

Mattering as a Psychosocial Concept

At first, we sought a synonym for mattering because we thought it might be perceived as a particularly unusual word. But, to our surprise, we learned that mattering is a recognized but relatively unstudied psychosocial concept, originating from Moos and Moos' (1976) social climate concept and initially described by Rosenberg and McCullough (1981). Flett (2018) in the subtitle of his comprehensive book referred to mattering as "The human need to be significant." He noted that there is a limited amount of research and theory on mattering, but it is a construct well worth studying because mattering is "something that matters to most people to some extent" (Flett, 2018, p. 5). Our goal, however, was not to study mattering per se, nor do we now wish to critique the concept or place ourselves in the field of community psychology, though it may be that our findings are useful for furthering the theoretical descriptions of mattering. But mattering arose as the output of our model of how EPPs interact with parents of children with CCCs, and so it is important to discuss. The literature on mattering only affirms the importance of this concept in our study:

> Whether we come to feel we matter or don't matter depends to a substantial degree on how other people interact with us. The quality and nature of our interpersonal experiences impact and shape our appraisals of mattering or not mattering.
>
> (Flett, 2018, p. 51)

Flett (2018) emphasized that mattering is central to people's lives and is based in the human need to feel connected to others: To be accepted and included, to be valued members of social groups, and to contribute positively to the lives of oneself and others. Mattering is highly applicable across geographic and cultural boundaries; it creates an atmosphere where diversity is valued rather than a source of friction. Emerging from Flett's work is the point that mattering is a vital psychological resource that, as a key facet of social well-being, is not only associated with less emotional distress but also links with multiple indicators of positive adjustment.

Mattering is a key resource factor that contributes to a heightened level of resilience in general, but especially when faced with interpersonal adversities and challenges—such as, we would offer, those faced by parents of children with CCCs, as well as by the PHCPs who care for them, particularly since mattering may also buffer the ever-present fear of death (George & Park, 2016).

Another community psychologist, Prilleltensky (2020), explained that mattering consists of two complementary experiences: Feeling valued and adding value to oneself and to others. When persons feel valued, they are recognized and appreciated as the persons they are. Feeling valued also means that a person's inherent desire to belong is met by being welcomed and included, leading to positive emotions such as happiness or calm and well-being. In contrast, feeling rejected, excluded, or ignored leads to negative feelings, for example, anxiety or loneliness, and threatens well-being. Belonging is both a protective mechanism and a means of flourishing. Finally, feeling valued provides a sense of dignity that Prilleltensky (p. 18) regarded as "the backbone of mattering." Dignity implies feeling worthy by being recognized, acknowledged, included, and also respected for who one is and what one knows. It means feeling equal to others and being treated with fairness. Feeling valued, however, is a necessary though insufficient condition for mattering. To matter, people need to also add value, that is, they must make a meaningful difference to themselves and to others.

Adding value reflects human needs for self-determination, self-efficacy, and meaning. Self-determination involves autonomy (behaving according to one's own values), competence (having the ability to perform certain actions grounded in knowledge), and relatedness (establishing meaningful and supportive connections with others). Self-efficacy pertains to the belief that persons can make a difference; believing that they can take actions according to their goals makes them resilient in the face of adversity. Meaning derives from the need to have a sense of purpose. When these needs are impeded, people feel that they do not matter. Opportunities to meet these needs are influenced by the environment, some characteristics of which are more conducive than others to mattering.

Prilleltensky (2020) further identified four sources of feeling valued: Self, relationships, work, and community, all of which are related and fluid. These four sources are also the arenas in which people add value. People must find a balance between valuing and adding value in each arena because they cannot rely on just one: "Other people may show care and attention toward us, but nothing matters unless we care for ourselves as well" (Prilleltensky, 2020, p. 22). As well, the four arenas are interconnected so that if a person focuses on one, it is at the expense of the others; for example, if a person focuses on adding value only to themselves while ignoring the well-being of others, the person cannot expect much caring in return. Finally, the benefits of feeling valued lead to adding value, which, in turn, leads back to feeling valued, thus creating an iterative cycle of mattering. Prilleltensky also noted that mattering requires certain moral values aligned with valuing the well-being of personal (self), relational (others), and communal (work and community) well-being. He stated that all three moral values are particularly important in today's world, where there is so much emphasis on individualism to the extent that people tend to ignore relational and communal well-being. In short, feeling valued and adding value in these three realms are preeminent human needs and motivations. But, as Flett (2018, p. 200) noted, "Unfortunately, there has been little consideration thus far of precisely what significant others actually do to convey to a person that he or she matters and what is effective in making someone feel like he or she matters." Our findings, based on what makes it possible for EPPs to create a milieu of mattering with parents of children with CCCs, offer some insights into what is required to convey mattering.

EPPs and Mattering With Parents

EPPs' personal, relational, and collective values are founded in their broad worldview in which they see humanity as deeply interdependent. Thus, EPPs perceive that everybody matters, that every person has value and deserves recognition and respect, that relationships are integral to meaningful interaction, and that those relationships are core to effective societal functioning. EPPs' worldviews incorporate seeing things as larger wholes, as complex systems, which allows EPPs to visualize individual parents within the contexts that matter to them—their family, culture, and diversity. EPPs' valuing of social justice and equity and their own personal integrity are also foundational in directing them to treat all parents fairly and respectfully, thus enabling parents' feelings of dignity, being noticed, and being valued—parents feel that they matter to EPPs. EPPs' sense of being committed to the overarching purpose of authentic interaction is essential in how they relate to parents on a human-to-human level, so not coming across as better than, superior to, or overly attached to their professional role and status, thus preventing the impression that they or their opinions matter more than the parents'. This is not to say that EPPs dismiss the value of their own position, knowledge, or skills; they acknowledge their abilities but see themselves not as heroes but as one of many who are involved and who matter in parents' lives.

Despite the breadth of their worldview/values and the depth of their purposeful commitment, EPPs are sensitive to and able to focus on the distinctiveness of each parent's particular situation. By orienting with every encounter, EPPs consistently make parents feel welcome not only in the place where their child is being cared for but as valued partners in the child's care. EPPs reinforce such parental responses when they seek parents' perspectives about the particularities of what matters most to them, thus giving parents visibility and a voice. EPPs' initial encounters with parents lay the groundwork for developing a relationship through which EPPs' interest in learning about what matters to parents generally—their hopes, fears, goals, interests, values, and thoughts about the current situation—leads to parents feeling that they are not being judged and that they matter as persons. Mattering is central to the formulation of real relationships between EPPs and parents—both will be engaged if they feel valued.

EPPs take into account what matters most to parents while discerning, shaping, and checking their own responses to parents. Because EPPs discern that parents have different needs and different perceptions of what matters most to them at a particular point in time, EPPs shape and check their behavior accordingly. When reflecting, EPPs consider if and how they attend to what matters most for parents and for themselves. Reflecting is a constant endeavor for EPPs and is closely related to self-awareness, that is, understanding who they are and how they are feeling at a particular moment is key to achieving authenticity and congruence between their intent and their actions. Without such personal knowledge, PHCPs are at risk of losing touch with themselves—and under such conditions, authenticity and congruence cannot be demonstrated. Such moments of reflection often require only a brief suspension of activity to focus their attention and create an interpersonal climate that enhances meaningful connections. All the while, EPPs' are responsive to what parents need at the moment, and they connect by listening, empathizing, suspending judgment, pacing, maintaining hope, focusing on the positive, showing kindness, and building trust—all of which contribute both to parents feeling that they matter and to the EPPs' sense of making a difference.

EPPs' desire for learning, their curiosity, their professional and general knowledge, and their competence are all part of fulfilling their human need to make a difference by mastering the environment so they can feel effective in adding value to their own lives and the lives of parents. Through empowering, EPPs treat parents as partners, believing that parents relish opportunities to learn new skills to make a difference in the direct care of their ill child. A milieu of mattering promotes parents' learning of skills that helps them to adapt to the pervasive uncertainty of having a child with a CCC. Using what they learn from EPPs' teachings and from observing EPPs' behavior, many parents support other parents in the unit, which leads to enhanced well-being and, thereby, feeling that they add value to those families. The dual nature of mattering (feeling valued and adding value) means that EPPs seek personal meaning and social harmony at the same time, thus supporting the idea that it is not possible to value others without first valuing oneself. By practicing self-care, EPPs find a balance between giving attention to themselves and to others. In Chapter 9 of his book, Flett (2018) extended the focus of mattering as a clinically relevant construct by considering the role of mattering in the therapeutic process, underscoring the fact that the feeling of mattering or not mattering is central to relational experiences. The harmonious, professional human-to-human relationship that develops between EPPs and parents is integral to developing a milieu of mattering between them. But the key to developing this milieu of mattering is not just their relationship; it is also the coming together of all the components of the process of attuning.

EPPs and Mattering at Work

When explaining their choice of a profession in health care, our PHCP participants often referred to their yearning to help others, reflecting a particular desire to positively influence others' lives. EPPs derive intrinsic benefits and meaning from helping children with CCCs and their parents: *When I think of what's rewarding for me and feeling satisfied with my work, or what I find most meaningful, it's when you have that human-to human meeting with an individual at their core and there's that connection.* EPPs feel valued by parents for the work that they do and feel that they add value to the lives of parents and their children. But EPPs also welcome being recognized, valued, and appreciated by the people with whom they work. As we noted earlier in Chapter 9, EPPs approach their team members and other colleagues in the same way they interact with parents—via the process of attuning. Guided by their worldview, it matters to EPPs that they can enact their values and commitment to authentic engagement with colleagues as well as with parents. And, as with parents, the result is an interpersonal milieu of mattering that evolves between EPPs and their colleagues and also extends to the team.

A milieu of mattering in a team is characterized by team members feeling that they have a place on the team—that they belong, that their coworkers perceive their contributions as significant and also appreciate them for their work and for the persons that they are. Leaders are particularly important in contributing to a milieu of mattering in their team, in the setting, and in the institution. Leaders who are EPPs themselves find ways of making others feel like they matter. For example, by developing one-on-one connections with each team member, these leaders learn what matters to each individual as a person. Team members then feel that they matter; they are not just a cog filling an empty slot on a rotation schedule. While regularly providing feedback to PHCPs about their work—if it was going well or if it needed to be tweaked, or advanced, or redirected—leaders do so in conversation where both the leader and the clinician have opportunities to engage in dialogue. This too makes PHCPs feel that they matter; they are inspired and guided about how to add even more value to the team's work.

Our model represents an iterative mattering cycle in which EPPs' approach to interaction with parents and their coworkers results in both groups feeling that they matter to the EPPs. Being appreciated by both groups, EPPs feel that they in turn matter to parents and coworkers. Each group is gratified that they make a difference in the lives of the other. Mattering reinforces EPPs' desire to continue to sustain their worldview, values, and ongoing commitment to authentic engagement: *It reinforces your values if the outcomes are good.* The more likely it then becomes that EPPs' influence extends to others in creating a milieu of mattering in their setting, their institution, and their broader society.

EPPs experience little or no burnout—something that they attribute to the milieu enabling them to practice according to their values and purpose even though their commitment requires considerable effort. They are clear that not practicing according to their values and purpose is the major source of burnout:

> That level of engagement and self-awareness and being in the moment every day, during every part of the day, during highs and lows, takes a lot of physical and mental output which is why I love doing what I do. I think that such hard work makes you less burnt out because if you're not practicing at that depth, or in line with how you envision how your practice should be, you know inside yourself that you're short-changing yourself and the families. I prefer to dive in full on because I know those rewards at the end of the day are there for the family and myself, every day.

EPPs identify that being short-staffed is really

> the cause of any burnout because you cannot do what you believe you should be doing. Sometimes I love that challenge of increasing technology. If we have enough staff on, it makes the difference but if we don't, that's when people get burned out because you don't get the time to spend with the family.

Similarly, in his chapter on work and mattering Flett (2018) noted that research in a variety of fields indicates that clinicians' sense of mattering to other people at work and to the overall institution contributes to job satisfaction, resilience, commitment, and less burnout. More recently, Haizlip and colleagues (2020), based on a cross-sectional survey of over 300 nurses in the United States, reported that higher levels of mattering at work were associated with lower burnout and higher engagement. EPPs are protected from burnout because they feel a sense of existential significance, that they themselves and what they do are useful and important; that their lives matter in the larger scheme of things.

Using the Model of Exemplary Interaction to Enact Person-Centered and Relational Care

Our model of exemplary interaction relates closely to the approaches espoused by proponents of person-centered care, an umbrella under which patient- and family-centered care fall, as well as by supporters of relational care. Such approaches advocate for how health care could be improved by providing care in certain ways, that is, by individualizing care for the person regardless of setting. Our model, however, operationalizes the concepts articulated in the person-centered and relational care approaches and offers concrete, actionable steps that health-care providers (HCPs) can take to improve the experience of care for both parents and themselves. Our model shows explicitly <u>how</u> to do what these other models advocate needs to happen. For example, each approach directs HCPs to treat others with dignity, assuming that it is an easy thing to do. However, our model makes explicit the personal characteristics that HCPs must develop to actually ensure that the dignity of others is recognized.

The literature is replete with articulations of patient-centered, family-centered, and relational care, many of whose authors bemoan the technological and bureaucratic emphases that create an impersonal, and sometimes inhumane, character of health care; they advocate for their particular approach as the way to counteract these troubling conditions. For example, the concept of patient-centered care was included in the landmark Institute of Medicine (US) Committee on Quality of Health Care in America (IOM; IOM, 2001) report, *Crossing the Quality Chasm: A New Health System for the 21st Century*, as one of the fundamental approaches to improving the quality of US health care. The IOM defined patient-centered care as being respectful of and responsive to individual patient preferences, needs, and values; care that ensures patient values guide all clinical decisions. This definition highlights the importance of clinicians and patients working together to produce the best possible outcomes via shared decision-making.

Similarly, family-centered care is an approach to the planning, delivery, and evaluation of health care that is grounded in mutually beneficial partnerships among HCPs, patients, and families; it first took hold in pediatrics, particularly in the care of children with long-term illness or disability. The Institute for Patient- and Family-Centered Care (www.ipfcc.org/) notes that in both patient-centered and family-centered care, patients and families define who constitutes their own family and determine how family will participate in care and decision-making. The core values of dignity, respect, information sharing, participation, and collaboration underlie patient- and family-centered care and the overall goal is to promote health and well-being. But implied in patient- and family-centered approaches is the centrality of how HCPs relate to or interact with patients and families; attention is not directed toward the abilities of the HCPs themselves in this regard. Yet, parents typically rate human qualities of clinicians (e.g., kindness, concern, sensitivity, approachability) as being of much higher importance than technical competencies. What seems to be forgotten by too many HCPs is that patients of all ages and conditions and, notably, parents of children with CCCs, indicate that their relationships with HCPs constitute a key factor in their satisfaction with care.

Despite the widely acclaimed implementation of patient-/family-centered care into many settings, many HCPs despair over the actual extent of such an approach into their settings. Our model focuses on what constitutes excellent PHCP-parent interaction, so by integrating it into patient-/ family-centered care and emphasizing the connection between clinicians and those they care for, our model can strengthen patient-/family-centered care and its impact.

A relationship-centered approach focuses more directly on the HCPs and what they bring to the caregiving situation. This approach focuses on "whatever transpires when the world of care seekers and the world of care providers meet and interact in a setting of care and community context" (Papadatou, 2009, p. 15). The relationship-centered approach acknowledges the subjective world of the care seeker (in our case, parent/child), of the PHCP, and of the other key persons who are directly or indirectly involved in the process (PHCP's coworkers, ill child's siblings, other family members), as well as the intersubjective space formed as a result of the encounter (milieu of mattering), the work and organizational context (setting and organization), and the community and sociocultural milieu in which the situation unfolds. "In fact, the relationship-centered approach is concerned with the development of large networks of relations among people, professionals, teams, and communities that have the potential to be caring, enriching, and rewarding for all parties involved" (Papadatou, 2009, p. 17). A relational consciousness extends clinicians' attention beyond the individual level to the relational level, which occurs at and between the intrapersonal, interpersonal, and contextual levels (Doane & Varcoe, 2015). This approach closely relates to our model of exemplary interaction in which we make visible the relational components of excellent interaction.

Also related to our model of exemplary interaction is the relational-based palliative approach that uses palliative care principles (e.g., dignity, hope, comfort, quality of life, relief of suffering) with people facing chronic, life-limiting conditions at all stages, not just at the end of life. It reinforces personal autonomy, the right for persons to be actively involved in their own care, and a greater sense of control for individuals and families. The palliative approach "does not closely link the provision of care with prognosis" (Stajduhar, 2011, p. 10); rather, it focuses (more broadly) on "conversations with patients/families about their needs and wishes" (Stajduhar, 2011, p. 10). In pediatrics, it aims to help parents and their children with CCCs have the fullest lives possible in the present, instead of sacrificing time now for time later. Within the field of pediatric palliative care, such conversations are a reality.

When asked, most PHCPs, like many other HCPs, can easily remember special moments of closeness with parents of ill children that were beneficial for both the parent and the clinician. Far from coincidental, these moments can offer instruction about the relational dimension of human experience that is integral to optimal pediatric care, particularly the care of children with CCCs and their parents. But some PHCPs, though well intentioned, lack explicit guidance about this dimension because their focus is directed solely to the objective assessment and management of clinical symptoms. If instead they were taught according to a biopsychosocial approach to health and healing that includes learning about relational care, inherent in which is learning about themselves, then our model of exemplary interaction could prove useful in teaching clinicians about the interconnectedness that predisposes to the feelings of mattering that are at the very heart of healing.

Further Thoughts on the Milieu of Mattering

Most PHCPs try to do the right thing at least most of the time. But in the world of increasing technology and bureaucratization, of increasing complexity and specialization, specialists within the system may become more and more focused on their own particular area of expertise—not through any fault of their own, but just because of how increasingly complex systems work, that is, moving toward entropy (disorder). Eventually, specialists may lose their sense of how their actions connect to what others—both colleagues in and outside of their own discipline, and parents—are doing. Despite their good intentions, working hard, and following the rules, they may become oblivious to any shortcomings that arise in social systems. EPPs, however, retain their sense of the whole and their commitment to engaging authentically with others. Thus, their interactions with parents of children with CCCs result in relationships that create a social environment where what matters to parents and what matters to the PHCPs is similar—a common interest in providing optimal care to children with CCCs. EPPs and parents feel both valued and that they add value to the situation. This environment, as with all natural or social environments, is constantly in flux and EPPs and parents alike must adapt to the changes while maintaining their commitment to what matters. Adaptation in a health-care setting almost always means taking all relevant values into account and cooperating with others. By working together, EPPs and parents learn ways of adapting to changes in the child's condition, within themselves, within the overall team, and in the institution and the society.

As an individual, you can learn how to develop and contribute to a milieu of mattering. We suggest you use the questions in Box 11.1 to help you consider what you might do to help you in your quest to provide the optimal milieu for your patients, their families, your colleagues, and yourself.

Throughout this book, we have tried to provide examples of how you can become, or continue to be, an EPP who interacts with patients, families, and colleagues in ways that maximize both their experience and your own potential. We have described our model of exemplary interaction and the various parts that comprise the model, from the importance of worldview, values, and commitments to the milieu of mattering. In the next, the final, chapter, we turn our attention to the broader implications of our model and offer our suggestions about how to move beyond the individual to taking actions that in a more systemic way can facilitate positive outcomes and optimal interaction in every setting.

Box 11.1: Milieu of Mattering: Questions for Consideration

- After going back to Chapter 3 and thinking about my own worldview, values, and commitment as I review the chapter, how do I think my worldview and so forth affect how I contribute to a milieu of mattering?
- After going back to Chapter 4 and reminding myself what attuning means, how do I think I enact the facets of attuning in my own work? What could I do to improve my practices?
- How do I show patients and their families that I value them? Respect them?
- After going back to Chapter 6 and reminding myself about connecting behaviors, how do I think I enact these connecting behaviors in my own work? What could I do to improve my practices?
- Do I feel that I am valued by the children I care for and their parents? Respected?
- What makes me feel valued by patients and parents? Respected? How could I practice in ways that might enhance my feelings of being valued and respected by patients and their parents?
- Do I value my colleagues? Respect them? How could I practice in ways that might enhance how I show that I value and respect colleagues?
- Do I feel that I am valued by my colleagues? Respected by them? How could I practice in ways that might enhance my feelings of being valued and respected by colleagues?
- What value do I contribute to my institution? To society? How could I increase my contributions so I increase my value?
- How do I think my potential for burnout might be affected by feeling that my life and my work matters?

References

Doane, G. H., & Varcoe, C. (2015). *How to nurse: Relational inquiry with individuals and families in changing health and health care contexts.* Wolters Kluwer.

Flett, G. (2018). *The psychology of mattering: The human need to be significant.* Academic Press.

George, L. S., & Park, C. L. (2016). Meaning in life as comprehension, purpose, and mattering: Toward integration and new research questions. *Review of General Psychology, 20*(3), 205–220. https://doi.org/10.1037/gpr0000077

Haizlip, J., McCluney, C., Hernandez, M., Quatrara, B., & Brashers, V. (2020). Mattering: How organizations, patients, and peers can affect nurse burnout and

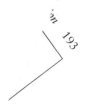

ursing Administration, 50(5), 276–273. https://doi.org/10.1097/
?

mmittee on Quality of Health Care in America. (2001).
w health system for the 21st century. National Academies
.26/10027

.. (1976). A typology of family social environments. *Family*
. 1. https://doi.org/10.1111/j.1545-5300.1976.00357.x

). *In the face of death: Professionals who care for the dying and the bereaved.*
.ishing.

.y, I. (2020). Mattering at the intersection of psychology, philosophy, and poli-
American Journal of Clinical Psychology, 65(1–2), 16–34. https://doi.org/10.1002/
.jcp.12368

Rosenberg, M., & McCullough, B. C. (1981). Mattering: Inferred significance and mental health among adolescents. *Research in Community & Mental Health, 2,* 163–182.

Stajduhar, K. I. (2011). Chronic illness, palliative care, and the problematic nature of dying. *Canadian Journal of Nursing Research, 43*(3), 7–15. https://cjnr.archive.mcgill.ca/article/download/2313/2307/0

12 Implications of the Model of Exemplary Interaction

If you were to use this model for teaching, it would give students a more comprehensive idea of communication as interaction. It's not just what you know or say, but how you say it—it's all these aspects of the windmill. It requires learning by doing, but not by doing one interaction—you need to watch hundreds of them, do hundreds of them; students always learning and teachers always modeling.

As we (the authors) learned back in graduate school, the "So what?" question is crucial to all research projects. It subsumes readers' potential questions: What does it all mean? What is its significance? Why does it matter? We noted in Chapter 11 that a milieu of mattering is the result of all the components of the model coming together. In this final chapter, we identify how and why our overall findings matter and describe implications derived from our study. The suggestions we offer may be neither unique nor all-inclusive, but they are congruent with our findings and have been validated by our participants and other HCPs beyond pediatric settings.

Meaning of Our Overall Findings

Our study was rooted in curiosity about why parents of children with CCCs noted that most interactions with PHCPs were good but only a few were excellent. When asked to describe what made those particular interactions stand out, parents replied that those PHCPs treated them as human beings. Thus, our aim was to identify what makes it possible for such PHCPs to engage optimally with parents of children with CCCs. Our resulting conceptualization provides empirical evidence that the interactions of PHCPs who are perceived by parents and other PHCPs as exemplary are rooted in an encompassing worldview and a commitment to authentic engagement with parents; founded in the depth and breadth of EPPs' knowledge, persistent curiosity, flexibility/open-mindedness, and self-awareness; and influenced by EPPs' past experience, their self-care, and the contexts within which encounters occur. Central to exemplary interaction is the process of exquisitely attuning to particularities of the situation in the present moment.

DOI: 10.4324/9780429352393-12

The coming together of all components creates a milieu of mattering in which both parents and EPPs feel that not only do they themselves matter but they also make a difference in each other's lives as partners in caring for children with CCCs. The windmill metaphor (see Figure 2.2, Chapter 2) illustrates how all the components fit together to create exemplary interaction. Our aim in this book was to render more visible the intricacies of what enables some PHCPs to engage in exemplary interactions with both parents and colleagues.

So, what do our findings mean? First, our focus on what PHCPs did well rather than on what was lacking shows not only that it is possible for PHCPs to interact in exemplary ways but also that those who do so are recognizable as excellent. Second, our findings indicate that EPPs provide the positive outcomes parents desire and give direction for parents who are eager to do their part in advocating for their child's care: *This model gives us as parents the words that we never had before to describe what we mean by excellence. It can help us speak up for what is missing or to commend the best providers.* Thus, the model both reinforces the parent's role in decision-making and explicates for PHCPs what is involved in relinquishing their role as a paternalistic authority so that they can become more effective coaches and partners. In other words, PHCPs can learn how to ask not only "What is the matter?" but also "What matters to you?"

Third, our study not only supports existing knowledge about the positive aspects of interactions between PHCPs and parents but also extends that knowledge by providing a comprehensive picture of the relationships between PHCPs and parents, as well as with coworkers. The model demonstrates that although most PHCPs can be very good in some aspects of the model, it is the purposeful, consistent, and simultaneous engagement in all components of the model that reflects exemplary practice and explains why only some PHCPs are perceived as exquisite practitioners.

Finally, it has previously been noted that "attempts to personalize medicine have not had much impact because no one knew well the traits lacking in medicine nor how to teach them" (Charon, 2006, p. 8). Our model now names these missing components of human-to-human interaction and, using a metaphorical windmill, clearly shows how they relate to one another, thus indicating how they can be taught and integrated into clinical practice. Moreover, by identifying and detailing the components of exemplary interaction, the findings counteract the common perception that excellence in interaction is simply a matter of personality.

Extrapolating Beyond Pediatric Settings

The link between encounters with HCPs and patient/family outcomes is not limited to pediatrics. A robust body of adult-focused literature has demonstrated positive associations between the patient experience of care and relevant clinical outcomes, including adherence to therapeutic regimens, health-care service use, and the safety of care delivery (Doyle et al., 2013; Price et al., 2014; Zolnierek & DiMatteo, 2009). Adult patients and their family members express satisfaction with providers who listen carefully to their concerns, demonstrate empathy, and make an effort to design care that incorporates the family's unique needs and preferences. More importantly, adult patients and families feel empowered to make changes to their health routines and to use supportive and cost-effective health resources when they have been active participants in the co-creation of their plan of care (Doyle et al., 2013). At the same time, more than half of surveyed patients and physicians believe the health-care system fails to consistently deliver compassionate care (Lown et al., 2011), suggesting that some of the costs and poor outcomes of care may be attributable to poor quality interactions with HCPs. A growing body of work in the field of adult care highlights the importance of the patient experience but fails to offer guidance on how best to engage with patients and families to foster a positive experience.

In the process of conducting our study, and particularly in our analysis discussions, we realized that our evolving conceptualization pertained to many of our own clinical experiences beyond children with life-threatening illness. We reflected on how most research with adult patients has focused on verbal communication and content rather than on the reciprocal influence of individuals on each other's behaviors, emotions, attitudes, and perceptions, both verbally and nonverbally, as well as the context of the interactions (Fine et al., 2010). We realized that examples from our data could have easily come from adult patients with a variety of conditions across multiple settings, as well as their family members, and that our data also mirrored comments from HCPs in settings other than pediatrics. In fact, some of the findings echoed results from our earlier studies in not only pediatrics but also adult settings (e.g., Davies et al., 1995; Davies & Oberle, 1990; Fitch & Steele, 2010a, 2010b; Steele & Fitch, 1996a, 1996b, 2008a, 2008b). We also found that we could easily identify with many of the situations in examples of encounters with HCPs in our own professional lives. As we neared completion of our initial conceptualization and returned to our three settings to seek input from participants and from expanded groups of HCPs, we received overwhelmingly positive input that verified our interpretation of the findings. We were told that the model fits perfectly with the experiences of the group members—not only in their pediatric work settings but in all other settings where they had worked as well.

We then began to present the conceptualization at conferences so that we could gain additional input and verify the findings on a broader scale. At the time of writing, we have given more than 30 presentations at a variety of conferences: locally, nationally, and internationally. Audiences have included not only clinicians and administrators but also practitioners from various fields, for example, bereavement counselors, psychologists, therapists, chiropractors, and chaplains. Educators, theologians, philosophers, and sociologists, as well as computer technicians and engineers, have also been part of some audiences. Their input mirrored that of our local setting audiences—the conceptualization fit for them and for the work that they did: *Your model is really more than a model for dealing with parents of an ill child; it is a model for living, for all of us.* Thus, although we now discuss implications that arose from a study within the context of pediatric care in urban settings, we want you to consider how these suggestions might be applicable in adult and other settings as well, such as in rural areas and in home care.

Implications of Our Findings for Professional Education

Given the influential role in our model of a broad worldview, its related values, and a commitment to authentic engagement, we pondered how to foster the development of these aspects—particularly in students but also for clinicians—within health-care disciplines. Professional education is, of course, not limited to the education that occurs in postsecondary institutions; HCPs are engaged in continuous learning throughout their careers to stay abreast of changes in practice and to learn new techniques for care delivery. Some health-care organizations offer continuing education opportunities to HCPs that can and should, but typically seldom do, include opportunities for staff to engage with and think critically about their practice. It is worthwhile considering if there could be ways for more HCPs to become exemplary clinicians. What if students in professional health-care programs, for example, medicine, nursing, and social work, or clinicians in pediatric settings, were selected with consideration of our model? What if schools and organizations recruited students and staff who identified with an expansive worldview and the values that underpin it? What if a change in how such students and clinicians were educated could help broaden their worldview and values, as well as their sense of commitment to human interaction?

Shifting the Goal of Higher or Professional Education

Before addressing these questions, it is relevant to consider how the goal of higher education has changed over time and how it may be time to circle round and incorporate some of the earlier goals into today's health-care education. Sociologist Chad Hanson (2014) noted that American higher education initially was patterned primarily after the Oxford and Cambridge universities in Britain, which held character formation as central to their mission. Then, in the early 20th century, the purpose began to move toward the German model that emphasized research and the production of knowledge. By 1970, the shift from teaching college to research university had unfolded and science- and technology-oriented fields became privileged. Hanson suggested that universities then abandoned the big questions about who their students become and no longer concentrated on the development of students as persons. During recent decades, postsecondary and professional schools have been seen as engines of economic development (Engell & Dangerfield, 2005); education is thought of as career preparation, and students are viewed, narrowly, as economic resources. Thinking of students as a human form of capital potentially means that "We run the risk of limiting ourselves to questions about what students know or how they perform prescribed tasks. We lose sight of the notion that schools allow people to forge new selves" (Hanson, 2014, p. 10).

Our study participants, particularly physicians but excluding social workers, commented on how little, if any, emphasis in their education was on their development as persons. During a Grand Rounds presentation about our model, a junior medical student asked with sincere curiosity about one of the facets of the model: *How does one become more self-aware?* Clearly, self-awareness as a concept had not yet received attention in his education; yet self-awareness is integral to reaching our full potential as human beings and as exemplary care providers. In our presentations, we also noted that some HCPs seemed to assume they were practicing as EPPs but, in fact, they were unaware of the impact of their interactions on others. Those who were actually EPPs were the most curious about how they could use the model to become even more effective in their interactions. We are fully aware of how many readers of this book might believe that self-exploration is unnecessary to their professional duties, that it is a waste of time and touchy feely, and not at all relevant to them, but we found that who EPPs are as people is central to their professional interactions and ability to engage authentically with parents. EPPs demonstrate that education is first and foremost about learning to develop the intellectual capacities needed to succeed as professionals and as human beings. In the end, it is not only a matter of <u>what</u> they do; it is <u>how</u> and <u>why</u> they do it and the knowledge required above all else is knowledge of yourself.

Participants also lamented the insufficient attention paid to person-to-person interaction skills in their educational programs. Many felt that they did not get knowledge about or experience with interacting with patients; they were thrown in the deep end and so made a lot of mistakes, especially at the start. Rather than ad hoc learning within their work settings, EPPs also desired more systematic continuing education and mentoring regarding how to interact more effectively with parents, because it is helpful for them to see other people interact with parents. They recognized that they have their own ways, but every time they see somebody else talk effectively to parents, they think, *Oh, that's a good way of expressing that idea.* Still, experienced HCPs may be challenged when changing their embedded patterns of interaction. Even Atul Gawande, a well-known practicing surgeon and author, confessed how in his career he was always most comfortable being Dr. Informative, the technical expert who let the patient, as consumer, make the decisions. But this approach was not helpful for many patients who preferred to have Dr. Interpretive, based on creating a partnership in which the doctor asked what is most important to the patient. Putting this new approach into practice is not easy: "I felt foolish to still be learning how to talk to people at this stage of my career" (Gawande, 2014, p. 207). Learning, however, is ongoing for EPPs who suggested that every few years clinicians should ask themselves questions such as: What does this situation mean to me now? What have I lost? What do I still have? What have I learned? How do I see my role now?

Just as students learn manual skills through practicing them, they also need to practice how to interact with others. We suggest that teachers give students opportunities to practice interaction skills from early in their programs. Sending medical or other students in right away to counsel grief-stricken patients is unacceptable; they first need to watch people in practice doing it. One avenue for laying a foundation for relational skills is for new students to visit with real patients to talk with them about their lived experience with illness, disability, dying, and grieving and then, using the model as a guide, discuss their interactions. Students could then explore basic values, thus increasing their awareness of individual values, stereotypes, and perceptions that will influence their practice. This focus on relational skills should continue into the clinical areas as students make their way through their programs. For example, EPPs remembered that as students they were often invited to observe a procedure that was new to them, such as an intubation on a tiny baby. The same should apply to interaction skills, for example, inviting students to observe a conversation about a difficult topic. Each experience should be followed by a discussion between the teacher and the student.

In too many cases the current supervisory model focuses on imparting information as a one-way process: Messages are delivered and assumed to be understood and incorporated, so students learn to tell, not talk with. Our model requires a more dialogical approach, which is so important because the focus of one's initial professional education/training sets a pattern that subsequently guides one's approach to patients. If there is no aspect of education early on that teaches students to see a larger relational picture (i.e., beyond the technical procedures), then the primary focus on the technical aspects consistently moves to the forefront. Our findings suggest that professional education must incorporate a focus on the development of HCPs' worldview, values, and commitment to authentic engagement, and all components of the model, so HCPs become not just professionals with valuable knowledge and prescribed skills but also considerate, compassionate individuals who can relate to others as fellow human beings. Attention must be paid in teaching and in clinical areas to the importance of taking time to pause, reflect, and take care of yourself. To this end, teaching about mindfulness is increasingly being included in various programs, such as the Mindful Medical Practice course at McGill University medical school (Hutchinson & Liben, 2020; Liben & Hutchinson, 2020). Students and HCPs need to understand the significance of spending time with patients/ families and a variety of people as a way of developing their worldview/

values and commitment. Further, making time for dialogue needs to be seen as a vital part of exemplary interaction rather than as something that takes time away from the more technical parts of practice.

Selecting Health-Care Students for Postsecondary Education

When selecting students for professional health-care educational programs, we suggest that it is important to start by seeking indicators of an expansive worldview in applicants. For example, have applicants list the countries they have visited and their volunteer community activities. Then, ask about the specific nature of their involvement and what lessons they learned from their experiences. Ask if applicants have a relative or friend who actively cared for others in the home or broader community, or if they themselves took a stand on issues of social justice or joined with family or others to work on projects that served the larger community. Ask about the role models and mentors they have had and what it was about those individuals that impressed them. Explore with applicants their connection with families, friends, or teams who are nearby and with people and places in faraway locations as an initial assessment of their perception of how diverse people, issues, and things are related. Ask questions about why they chose to apply for this particular program. Such questions would encourage prospective students to describe how they view the world and their values, how they engage with others who are different from them in some way, and where they stand with regard to an internal moral compass, for example, whether or not they are self-aware and can identify the importance of integrity.

Such questions would also facilitate assessment of an applicant's emotional intelligence (EI), a concept developed by Goleman (1995) in his book, *Emotional Intelligence*, in which he also summarized the importance of the emerging body of research on human emotion and its relationship to excellence. Emotionally intelligent individuals are both highly conscious of their own emotional states and able to identify and manage them; they are especially tuned in to the emotions of others. It is understandable that a sensitivity to emotional signals, both from within themselves and from their social environment, could contribute to EPPs' abilities for exemplary interaction. Our findings suggest that when deciding who should be admitted to health-care programs, EI is as important, if not more so, for developing a commitment to authentic engagement than emphasizing mostly GPAs and other forms of performance indicators. EI continues to be studied, first in fields such as human resources and organizational behavioral psychology, and in more recent years, within health-care professions where researchers have consistently shown that higher EI scores tend to be associated with positive findings, for example, more effective leadership, less burnout, higher clinical competence, and higher annual average academic grade (Dganit & Grinberg, 2018). These researchers also support our view that EI testing should be part of admission processes.

Selecting Clinicians for Health-Care Settings

Similarly, health-care settings should seek out potential employees who demonstrate a commitment to the values of diversity, social justice, family-centered care, and personal and professional integrity and who articulate a worldview consistent with those values and with the concept of authentic engagement. Interviews for clinical positions often revolve around discussion of the applicant's relevant professional experience and the ways in which they might handle complex clinical scenarios, but less attention is typically paid to investigating how applicants think about the world and how they understand and work with those different from themselves, whether patients, patients' families, or colleagues. Administrators hiring new team members can capture insights into applicants' worldview and values from the stories they tell, for example, when invited to share meaningful clinical interactions or scenarios in which conflict arose among colleagues. Listening for the worldview that informs an applicant's narrative can help managers to discern the applicant's commitment to authentic engagement with patients, families, and colleagues and their capacity for self-reflection and humility in interactions with others. Applicants can also be asked to respond to case scenarios that focus less on clinical management of the patient's condition and more on engagement in the interpersonal dynamics of the scenario. The applicant's response can similarly provide insight into their worldview and may help to highlight ways in which this worldview aligns or fails to align with the setting's or hiring unit's mission and values.

Teaching, Supervising, and Mentoring Students/Clinicians

We propose that educators, managers, and other clinical leaders need to be role models, mentors, and supervisors from whom students and clinicians can learn to practice according to the model. EPPs demonstrate a way of being in the world that underpins their interactions—so how do we teach students and clinicians a new way of being in the world?

Once accepted into their initial health-care program, students will be affected by the environment of the school, their particular program, and affiliated hospitals and other clinical facilities. The clinical environment also affects how clinicians engage in ongoing learning. Researchers have suggested that the scholastic environment contributes to what students learn (Thomson et al., 2017); our findings suggest that a milieu of mattering makes a difference for students' learning. Students have a strong desire to belong, a need that teachers can meet by applying the model to their interactions with students. First, teachers must examine their own worldview, values, and ways of being in the world. They must consider the depth of their commitment to authentic engagement with students. Teachers must listen to the students' perspectives by asking questions such as "What was that like for you?" "Can you tell me more about that?" and "What are you experiencing?" so that students feel heard, validated, and understood, that they and their ideas, thoughts, and questions matter. Teachers must discern what matters to students in the moment and shape their responses accordingly, check with and follow up with students, and, above all, reflect with them on their personal contributions to the interaction and on themselves while accepting their emotional responses without judgment but with honesty. Scaffolding reflective and interpersonal experiences with academic material helps students learn systems thinking and self-directed learning. If teachers model exemplary interactions with students, then together they create inclusive social spaces characterized by conditions of respect and dignity—the conditions necessary for developing a milieu of mattering, a sense of belonging. Classrooms and clinical encounters then become safe places for students to share their lives with each other and find support for integrating their cognitive academic learning and their emotional professional and personal growth and development.

By their ways of being hospitable to students and the dialogue that occurs between educators and students, professional schools can promote a worldview that includes values of inclusion, respect, accountability, fairness, and compassion and play a significant role in enabling students to learn that this is how we do things. Efforts of faculty, preceptors, and mentors to recognize students as individual persons and to work with them toward common goals can establish trust and have lifelong influence on students' worldview, values, and sense of commitment.

Clinicians too are affected by the environment in which they work. When setting and institutional leaders focus on attending to the range of human needs rather than on repairing bodies, there is greater opportunity to learn to practice as EPPs. When clinicians are made to feel welcome, they feel they matter and are, in turn, enabled to be inspirational mentors who create meaningful mentoring relationships with eager clinicians. For a good mentoring relationship to work, clinicians need to have a genuine connection with the mentee; they do not need to know everything, they just have to be real about what they know and do not know. Health-care settings have a responsibility to offer ongoing support and mentorship through all phases of an HCP's career. This mentorship can foster inquisitiveness among HCPs and can help to nurture a worldview that values continuous learning and self-reflection. During the vulnerable immediate post-licensure phase, this mentorship may be formal and frequent. Newly graduated nurses, for example, benefit from formalized mentorship experiences that help to normalize the challenges of a steep clinical learning curve and that provide a safe space for reflection on challenging interactions with patients, families, and colleagues (Van Patten & Bartone, 2019; Zhang et al., 2016). Once the learning curve has stabilized and the clinicians have moved beyond the new graduate phase, mentorship may be less formal and less frequent, with a stronger focus on development of the whole professional self. Settings that support this ongoing mentorship can help to foster the development of a professional workforce that is motivated to engage in continuous learning and that stays engaged and inquisitive about how to provide increasingly more sophisticated and more sensitive care to patients and families.

Students learn from a well-designed curriculum that not only addresses the necessary disciplinary content but also includes experiences that expand their worldview and values. Our model supports the idea that, in addition to a discipline-specific curriculum, students ought to complete more general courses to help further develop their worldview and values. For example, courses in the humanities might expose students to areas as diverse as music, theater, and art to literature, languages, and philosophy that offer different ways of considering humanity. Social science courses, including disciplines such as sociology, psychology, and anthropology, would also contribute to students' study of the human condition and, thus, expand students' understanding of their world. We also highly recommend well-planned curricular opportunities to learn about, and with, others who are different from themselves. Students may come to professional schools having studied diversity or cultures in various courses, but professional education must provide students with experiences that enable them to come to know those who are different from themselves as real people who live in a world both similar to and legitimately different from their own—especially in their own community. This is particularly true for students from majority populations who may not have previously engaged with individuals (patients, families, as well as colleagues) they will encounter within the realm of health care.

This learning should not be limited to the formal education setting but should instead extend into the clinical workplace. Increasingly, health-care organizations are recognizing a need to offer education that moves beyond the standard cultural competence curriculum to help clinicians engage with and understand concepts such as structural inequality, implicit bias, and the social determinants of health, all of which help to deepen clinicians' appreciation of and attentiveness to the unique challenges that individuals and families face as they navigate the health-care system and the broader community in which they live.

Creating opportunities for engaging in more subtle forms of difference—such as across health-care disciplines by having medical, nursing, and social work students and clinicians learn together in a shared environment—enables gaining an appreciation for each discipline's contribution to health care and lays the foundation for engaging in teamwork as practicing professionals. At the beginning of their professional degree programs, students could be required to participate in an interdisciplinary (at least nursing, medicine, and social work) seminar about the complexity of HCP–patient–parent/family interactions. The seminar would focus on the conceptualization of the components of exemplary interaction. Given that practical application is needed for students to engage beyond just the theoretical, students could be assigned into pairs or small groups with a mixture of disciplines and during the course they could learn from a particular patient/family chosen from a wide range of ages, conditions, locations of care, and family types. Weekly seminar discussions would focus on a different component of the model. Students could give feedback to their group members and other students, plus receive feedback, as a way of learning how to relate to patients and family members as persons. Practicing clinicians could also benefit from inter-professional discussion about their practice.

Engaging students and clinicians together in community activities where they have an opportunity to make a difference and can see their teachers and/or colleagues making a difference in the lives of people can reinforce a commitment to authentic engagement. Some professional programs already provide such experiential opportunities, for example, providing foot care in homeless shelters or spending a clinical placement in other geographic regions within their own country or in other countries. There are many areas that remain to be explored and that could expose students to opportunities for expanding their worldviews. Many health-care organizations sponsor community benefit activities, ranging from car seat checks to cardiopulmonary resuscitation training, and encourage their staff to volunteer for these programs. Doing so helps HCPs to better understand the community that they serve and often helps to reinforce or reconnect them to the reasons they became an HCP in the first place.

Regardless of discipline, ongoing development of the skills inherent in exemplary interaction must continue throughout the educational curriculum and into the professional practice setting. Based on our study, we suggest that one way to enhance interaction skills is to consider the tenets of narrative medicine (Charon, 2001, 2006; Frank, 2004), a shift away from the tendency to view the patient's story only through the lens of the biomedical model. Narrative competence involves seeing the patient's health issue(s) from their perspective and understanding their suffering. From the medical perspective, the story often ends with reaching the diagnosis, but for parents of children with CCCs, the story changes over time and requires that PHCPs listen to the ongoing narrative. Narrative medicine is complementary to evidence-based medicine; the narrative builds the bridge connecting, for example, the scientific evidence of clinical trials to the individual patient. Physicians who practice with both scientific and narrative competence are reported to be more empathetic, more resilient, find greater meaning in their work, and are less likely to burn out. It also leads to greater patient satisfaction (Kalitzkus & Matthiessen, 2009).

Narrative medicine would be a way of teaching values, commitment, reflection, and self-awareness. Adopting the methods of narrative competence, including reflective writing that should be reinforced as integral to students and clinicians' professional lives, means they could learn how to attend to patients' stories not as an instance of something that is universally true, but as a singular and meaningful situation and, consequently, develop their skills in attuning, connecting, and engaging in authentic dialogue. Moreover, patient storytelling when encouraged and listened to by HCPs is central to patients' healing (Charon, 2006).

In professional programs, specific courses could be explored to determine where discussion about the model and/or any of its components could best take place because students or clinicians cannot practice what they do not know. As with any skill, interaction skills require practice. For example, students could be reminded in skills laboratories that though technical skills are important, how they interact with the patient is equally as important. Educators could role model how to interact with a patient who is being started on intravenous antibiotics, and then students could be evaluated on how they demonstrate both their technical and their interactional skills. We suggest that students in courses where the profession is examined would benefit from discussion about the model and how to strive for exemplary practice. Other courses in which the model could be useful include courses about ethics, for example, the model could be used when discussing values clarification to emphasize the importance of HCPs understanding both their own values and the values of their patients. Or when discussing issues of justice, such as fair distribution of resources, the students could explore their own biases, assumptions, and values. We believe that there are many ways in which worldview, values, and commitment can (and should) be incorporated into the education of health-care students.

Using Our Model for Quality Improvement Purposes

Health-care settings typically conduct ongoing quality improvement initiatives as they seek to provide optimal care to patients and families, as well as sustain supportive work environments for employees. We suggest that fostering a milieu of mattering may be a mechanism by which organizations can achieve improvements in patient care delivery and employee engagement. For example, when parents feel comfortable with the team providing care to their child, they are more likely to speak up when they notice something wrong, offer feedback about how best to provide care for their child, or share concerns about caring for their child at home. This advocacy and partnership helps to create a safer environment for care that can, in turn, result in reductions in medical error rates or help to prevent avoidable re-admissions. Knowing that they matter to the team, parents are more likely to reflect positively on their hospital experience, which can translate into higher patient/parent satisfaction scores. Although currently not well tracked in most health-care settings, this sense of mattering may also translate into improvements in parental well-being that can both directly and indirectly impact the child's health and well-being.

In a milieu of mattering, EPPs too are better able to share their thoughts and observations and to ask questions, thus creating a psychologically safe environment that also translates into physical safety for patients and families. EPPs can more easily share their grievances in a way that is supportive, resulting in increased effectiveness, satisfaction, and productivity. EPPs working in a milieu of mattering find their relationships sustaining: They feel neither drained nor depleted; instead, they feel affirmed and stronger. EPPs who feel that they matter—that they are part of a team that cares about their well-being and is high functioning—are likely to report higher employee engagement scores and lower burnout levels and rates of job turnover. EPPs also recognize the positive impacts on the quality of care that result from an environment where everyone—patients, parents, and staff—matters, and these perceptions of safety may be captured on the safety culture assessments that many institutions periodically administer.

Flett (2018) devoted a full chapter to measuring mattering, describing various mattering measures and noting their reliability, validity, and potential for use in various situations. He indicated that developments in measurement will serve to further highlight the importance and relevance of the mattering construct. We too suggest that mattering is an important concept that deserves inclusion within quality improvement measurement.

Using Our Model to Combat Emergent Issues Within Health-Care Systems

When we started to write this book, we referred to the sorry state of the world and how it seemed that it might be increasingly difficult to be human. Now, as we come to the end of our writing, our world is in even more dire straits with the devastation wrought globally by COVID-19, a novel disease caused by the severe acute respiratory syndrome coronavirus 2 (SARS-CoV-2). Though vaccination programs have started, particularly in developed countries, global vaccination will take years. We are living with the horror of hundreds of millions of people who are sick, many of whom are ending up with challenging and chronic conditions post-infection, and over 4.5 million people have died. Our reality shows that the pre-existing disparities in health-care systems, even in supposedly advanced countries, have only been exacerbated by this pandemic. The people who are being hit the hardest are people of color, those who have lower levels of education, people who earn lower incomes than average, and those who are 70 years of age and older, especially if they live in communal settings such as nursing homes. Social injustices have been highlighted and no longer can be hidden. Vast improvements are needed to health-care systems to ameliorate the existing disparities and to prevent future disparities. We have witnessed how the response to COVID-19 has underscored the inhumanity of political leaders who ignored the experienced advice of public health leaders and we have seen how other leaders have done all they possibly could to fight the virus. We need people who understand exemplary interaction, who support justice for all, and who can be leaders in these challenging times; we need EPPs.

The pandemic has placed enormous pressure on health-care settings, clinicians, staff, and the health-care system at large. The isolation of patients from their families and the distancing of people in general from their friends, family members, and other social/work groups have created an epidemic of loneliness and mental health problems. COVID-19 has shown too clearly how contextual aspects can influence HCP interactions with their patients. The allocation and resourcing of personal protective equipment (PPE) has dominated conversations and decision-making. The scarcity of PPE has often made HCPs feel that they do not matter. Many families are frantic because they are not allowed to be with loved ones in care homes or hospitals, even when someone is dying. Many HCPs have become discouraged; they despair of being able to provide excellent care to their patients and families. The use of masks has been challenging because facial expressions are no longer a fairly easy way of gauging someone's demeanor or needs. The constant dealing with death has taken a serious toll on HCPs.

Yet some nurses, physicians, and so forth have found creative ways of trying to improve the situation, even if only a little bit. Short debriefing sessions at the end of shifts might include sharing one thing that made you smile today or where you felt you made a difference, which can boost morale and strengthen a feeling of mattering within the team. Masks might be partially covered with a photograph of the HCP so that the patient can see who is caring for them. It has been clear from television, radio, social media, and print sources that interaction and being human are critical to finding something good during this terrible pandemic. Various HCPs have talked about the importance of having families involved in decision-making and of how staff learn about the patient from the family. HCPs have told journalists about how of course staff need to express their emotions about the situation, that staff too are human, and that patients need to be treated as fellow human beings. We have been so proud of the many HCPs who have shown by their words and actions that they are EPPs, that they are doing their very best in challenging circumstances to still practice their commitment to authentic engagement with all patients and families, as well as with their colleagues. We have proudly witnessed the many ways in which HCPs are trying to make things at least a little bit better through their creativity and their commitment. And nightly 7 p.m. pot-banging that has rung out in support of these frontline workers is further evidence that the world values—and needs—EPPs. The time is right to change current health-care systems for the better. Our model of exemplary interaction provides one blueprint for moving forward.

Conclusion

And so we come to the end of our book. It has been an amazing experience for us to work together, and we all have grown and changed through the years it has taken to create something that is dear to our hearts. We leave you with us in transition as we shift from our regular biweekly book-writing meetings to other exciting endeavors. We hope that you too see yourself as in a transition—not at an end but at a new beginning as you start, or continue, your journey to being an exemplary practitioner in whatever area you choose to work. We hope that the ideas in our book not only have made you think and reflect on your own practice, on your own way of being in the world, of being a HCP, but they also have touched and inspired you. We know that EPPs' experience of joy in doing their work comes because of their pleasure in doing something that is better than it has to be; they are making good care even better. We hope that this too will be your experience. As we suggested earlier in the book, the use of our model of exemplary interaction is only limited by your own imagination—spread your wings and fly as you imagine the possibilities of your amazing career in health care!

References

Charon, R. (2001). Narrative medicine: A model for empathy, reflection, profession and trust. *Journal of American Medical Association, 286*(15), 1897–1902. https://doi.org/10.1001/jama.286.15.1897

Charon, R. (2006). *Narrative medicine: Honoring the stories of illness.* Oxford University Press.

Davies, B., Chekryn Reimer, J., Brown, P., & Martens, N. (1995). *Fading away: The experience of transition for families with terminal illness.* Baywood.

Davies, B., & Oberle, K. (1990). Dimensions of the supportive role of the nurse in palliative care. *Oncology Nursing Forum, 17*(1), 87–94.

Dganit, S., & Grinberg, K. (2018). Does the level of emotional intelligence affect the degree of success in nursing studies? *Nurse Education Today, 64*(5), 21–26. https://doi.org/10.1016/j.nedt.2018.01.030

Doyle, C., Lennox, L., & Bell, D. (2013). A systematic review of evidence on the links between patient experience and clinical safety and effectiveness. *BMJ Open, 3*(1), 1–18. https://doi.org/10.1136/bmjopen-2012-001570

Engell, J., & Dangerfield, A. (2005). *Saving higher education in the age of money.* University of Virginia Press.

Fine, E., Reid, M. C., Shengelia, R., & Adelman, R. D. (2010). Directly observed patient-physician discussions in palliative and end-of-life care: A systematic review of the literature. *Journal of Palliative Medicine, 13*(5), 595–603. https://doi.org/10.1089/jpm.2009.0388

Fitch, M., & Steele, R. (2010a). Identifying supportive care needs of women with ovarian cancer. *Canadian Oncology Nursing Journal, 20*(2), 66–74. https://doi.org/10.5737/1181912x2026674

Fitch, M., & Steele, R. (2010b). Supportive care needs of individuals with lung cancer. *Canadian Oncology Nursing Journal, 20*(1), 15–22. https://doi.org/10.5737/1181912x2011522

Flett, G. (2018). *The psychology of mattering: The human need to be significant.* Academic Press.

Frank, A. W. (2004). *The renewal of generosity: Illness, medicine and how to live.* University of Chicago Press.

Gawande, A. (2014). *Being mortal: Medicine and what matters in the end.* Metropolitan Books and Henry Holt and Company.

Goleman, D. (1995). *Emotional intelligence: Why it can matter more than IQ.* Bantam Books.

Hanson, C. (2014). Changing how we think about the goals of higher education. *New Directions for Higher Education, 2014*(166), 7–13. https://doi.org/10.1002/he.20090

Hutchinson, T. A., & Liben, S. (2020). Mindful medical practice: An innovative core course to prepare medical students for clerkship. *Perspectives on Medical Education, 9,* 256–259. https://doi.org/10.1007/s40037-020-00591-3

Kalitzkus, V., & Matthiessen, P. F. (2009). Narrative-based medicine: Potential, pitfalls, and practice. *Permanente Journal, 13*(1), 80–86. https://doi.org/10.7812/tpp/08-043

Liben, S., & Hutchinson, T. A. (2020). *MD aware: A mindful medical practice course guide.* Springer International.

Lown, B. A., Rosen, J., & Marttila, J. (2011). An agenda for improving compassionate care: A survey shows about half of patients say such care is missing. *Health Affairs, 30*(9), 1772–1778. https://doi.org/10.1377/hlthaff.2011.0539

Price, R. A., Elliott, M. N., Zaslavsky, A. M., Hays, R. D., Lehrman, W. G., Rybowski, L., Edgam-Levitan, S., & Cleary, P. D. (2014). Examining the role of patient experience surveys in measuring health care quality. *Medical Care Research and Review, 71*(5), 522–554. https://doi.org/10.1177/1077558714541480

Steele, R., & Fitch, M. (1996a). Coping strategies of family caregivers of home hospice patients with cancer. *Oncology Nursing Forum, 23,* 955–960.

Steele, R., & Fitch, M. (1996b). Needs of family caregivers of patients receiving home hospice care for cancer. *Oncology Nursing Forum, 23,* 823–828.

Steele, R., & Fitch, M. (2008a). Supportive care needs of women with gynecologic cancer. *Cancer Nursing: An International Journal for Cancer Care, 31*(4), 284–291. https://doi.org/10.1097/01.NCC.0000305743.64452.30

Steele, R., & Fitch, M. (2008b). Why patients with lung cancer do not want help with some needs. *Supportive Care in Cancer, 16*(3), 251–259. https://doi.org/10.1007/s00520-007-0301-4

Thomson, R., Docherty, A., & Duffy, R. (2017). Nursing students' experiences of mentorship in their final placement. *British Journal of Nursing, 26*(9), 514–521. https://doi.org/10.12968/bjon.2017.26.9.514

Van Patten, R. R., & Bartone, A. S. (2019). The impact of mentorship, preceptors, and debriefing on the quality of program experiences. *Nurse Education in Practice, 35*(2019), 63–68. https://doi.org/10.1016/j.nepr.2019.01.007

Zhang, Y., Qian, Y., Wu, J., Wen, F., & Zhang, Y. (2016). The effectiveness and implementation of mentoring program for newly graduated nurses: A systematic review. *Nurse Education Today, 37*(2016), 136–144. https://doi.org/10.1016/j.nedt.2015.11.027

Zolnierek, K. B. H., & DiMatteo, M. R. (2009). Physician communication and patient adherence to treatment: A meta-analysis. *Medical Care, 47*(8), 826–834. https://doi.org/10.1097/MLR.0b013e31819a5acc

Index

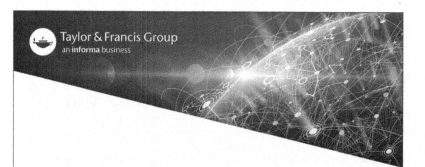

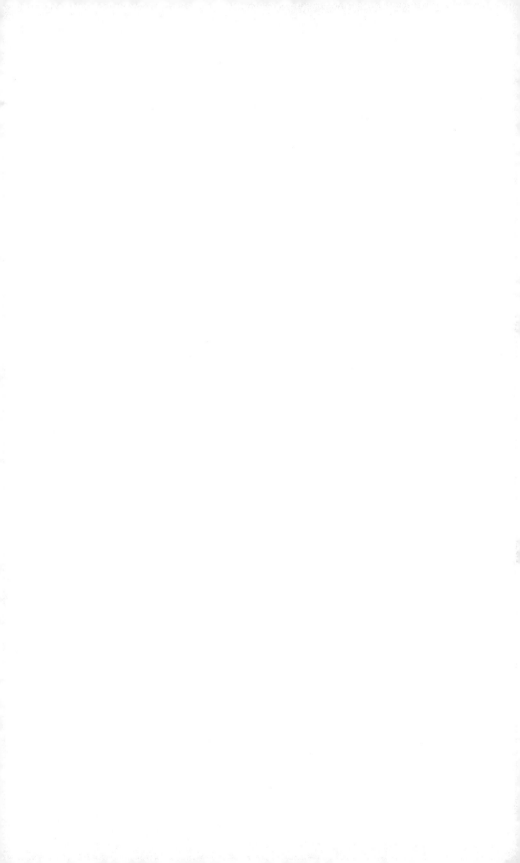